NO TIME TO CARE

A Leadership Game Plan to Ensure Caregiver Engagement

Charles Kunkle, RN MSN, CEN, NEA-BC

Published by Richter Publishing LLC www.richterpublishing.com

Editors: Monica San Nicholas, Mandi Weems & Diana Fisler

Formatted by: Monica San Nicholas

ISBN:0692614141
ISBN-13:9780692614143

REVIEWS

Insightful, Informative & Entertaining
Every once in a while you stumble upon a speaker who truly knocks your socks off. Charles Kunkle is one of those guys. As a healthcare insider, he knows the ins and outs of operations but it's his passion for service and patient engagement that makes him a standout on stage. His message is powerful and his delivery is impeccable. He has the timing of standup comedian and the insight of a compassionate healthcare veteran. The combination has his audiences laughing, crying and re-engaging with a stronger sense of purpose.
Kristin Baird, President/CEO
Baird Group

"I love this book. Drawing on his rich experiences as an E.R. nurse, dynamic leader and vibrant personality, Charles Kunkle brings terrific stories, humor and concrete tools together to provide a "How-to" guide to employee engagement. His ideas and insights can help all of us develop spirited and harmonious teams--- with employees who feel pride in their work and relationships and bring vibrancy and loving kindness to the patients and families they serve."
Wendy Leebov, Ed.D.
Language of Caring, LLC

As a board member of the Beryl Institute I was asked to introduce Charles Kunkle prior to his breakout presentation for the 2014 Beryl Conference. I had no prior knowledge of him or his work but immediately took notice when he began to speak, as he took the audience on a rollercoaster ride of emotions as his presentation unfolded. His in depth knowledge of the clinical world coupled with his emotional intelligence was clear as he captivated the audience with real life stories, analogies and humor that was unforgettable. The room was packed beyond capacity and all the buzz when he was done said, "Charles Kunkle was the best speaker of the entire conference!"
Colleen Sweeney RN, BS,
founder/owner of Sweeney Healthcare Enterprises

DISCLAIMER

This book is designed to provide information on healthcare. This information is provided and sold with the knowledge that the publisher and author do not offer any legal or medical advice. In the case of a need for any such expertise, consult with the appropriate professional. This book does not contain all information available on the subject. This book has not been created to be specific to any individual's or organization's situation or needs. Every effort has been made to make this book as accurate as possible. However, there may be typographical and/ or content errors. Therefore, this book should serve only as a general guide and not as the ultimate source of subject information. This book contains information that might be dated and is intended only to educate and entertain. The author and publisher shall have no liability or responsibility to any person or entity regarding any loss or damage incurred, or alleged to have incurred, directly or indirectly, by the information contained in this book. You hereby agree to be bound by this disclaimer or you may return this book within the guarantee time period for a full refund. In the interest of full disclosure, this book contains affiliate links that might pay the author or publisher a commission upon any purchase from the company. While the author and publisher take no responsibility for the business practices of these companies and or the performance of any product or service, the author or publisher has used the product or service and makes a recommendation in good faith based on that experience. All characters appearing in this work are fictitious. Any resemblance to real persons, living or dead, is purely coincidental.

DEDICATION

To my beautiful children, Grace and Jake, who have showed me the true meaning of love and given me an everlasting supply of laughter and joy.

To my mother, who showed me unconditional love and that I was able to be anything I wanted to be.

To my father, who helped me to understand the importance of respect and discipline and kept me on the straight and narrow as a young man.

To my many mentors, who have given me the tools to be the best leader possible for the bedside caregivers and the patients we have the honor to serve.

CONTENTS

I was sent the following poem by a very proud father. It was written by a 16-year old girl who was asked to write a spoken word poem for a class project. As I read it, it reminded me of the reason why I went into healthcare: to care for all people, rich or poor, old or young, gravely ill or mentally distressed. We are in the business of caring for human beings, not patients. This poem comes from the mind of a young woman who feels that at the age of 16 she has already seen the heartless, uncaring side of society. Think about the poem when you're in front of a difficult family member or that homeless man seeking medical care on a very cold day. Look for the 2.5 percent in everyone and you will once again transform your practice into what healthcare is supposed to be...a compassionate, healing environment.

CENTS

The modern penny is made of 97.5 percent zinc and 2.5 percent copper. Deemed cheaper and less worthy, the copper is masked behind the more valuable zinc as the two seemingly dissimilar elements are placed into the mighty Melting Pot, ultimately mass-producing a grand total of 7 billion individual pennies. But what is a penny worth if it has no means to express itself? We live in a world where a man's sense is defined by how many cents he has in his wallet; where only those more wealthy or better connected are elected to have an opinion, but what kind of a world do we live in that makes a man pay for the price of his own thoughts? Do not let them define your worth by your pocket size. Pennies—found tossed carelessly into the streets, rolling, staggering down dark alleyways, and wedged in-between pairs of worn out park benches. The lonely 2.5 percent are found roaming the streets, clad in tattered, urine-stained rags. Growing mad with their unheard thoughts of individuality, they beg for morsels of worth, and in return are stripped of their dignity and blamed for their improper use of the opportunities promised by the high-standing dollar. Today's Currency leaves man's mind left behind to rust and become oxidized with the polluted factory smoke, constantly pumped into the precious pulmonary veins of a mindless population while the mindful are treated—their privilege from conception—and taught that their affluence ascertains to the abundance of their wealth and that that wealth defines the value of the individualistic idea. But these blinders limit us from seeing what is happening underneath every zinc-gilded, heads-up penny that you pass on the streets.

Mackenzie Kunkle

PREFACE

I've been working in healthcare for more than 20 years. It seems like just yesterday that I walked onto that telemetry floor as a new nurse, excited about the opportunity to practice medicine, and at the same time, praying that I wouldn't kill anyone.

A lot has changed since then. I recall that as a new nurse I had the opportunity to sit at my patient's bedside and ask about their grandchildren or perhaps ask a military veteran about their time serving this great country of ours. I had the opportunity to make that human connection. Patient's were more than just a diagnosis. We had the opportunity to focus our care not only on the clinical component of care but on the human part as well.

Those times are gone. Healthcare reform, government regulatory changes and the focus on reducing costs has changed the healthcare landscape. Administrators are challenged to keep up with increasing government regulation and insurance company demands. As a healthcare leader, change seems to be ever present.

Those choosing healthcare now come to our doors educated and prepared with data that they have accessed from the internet. Numerous sites post our quality measures and patient satisfaction scores and allow the public to compare. To make it easy for consumers, the government has started assigning grades, in the way of stars, similar to the scoring system you use to pick a hotel or buy an item on Amazon. Healthcare is now a business.

We must adapt. We must overcome the hurdles and hardships to find ways to deliver patient care at reduced costs while maintaining the same quality and compassion. The future will be challenging, and as leaders, we must understand that we cannot do this alone. We will need to rely on the bedside caregiver to be open to new ideas, find creative solutions to new challenges, and continue to ensure that the focus of everything that we do stays on creating the ultimate patient experience.

Healthcare leaders have hired consultants and have adopted national programs to help them navigate this challenging new environment. Hourly rounding, bedside reports, and medication reconciliation are just some of the responsibilities that have fallen upon the shoulders of our bedside caregivers. Each requirement adding more to their already busy day. Is it any wonder that they have lost their ability to provide compassionate personal care? I was told by one caregiver that she felt like a task oriented zombie, shuffling from one room to another trying to complete the multiple tasks that she is required to complete in her 12 hour shift.

As leaders, we are asked to hold the bedside caregivers accountable to the target goals and metrics, and if unsuccessful, add more to their day in order to help "get us to the goal". We post graphs and target metrics on the billboard and send out dashboard reports for all to see. If you are honest with yourself, do you really think the bedside caregiver cares about that goal or graph? The constant reminders that they are not meeting the goal only frustrates them, which leads to discontent and discourages workers who only do the minimum required to survive the shift.

Do you think this approach is working? It's not about the numbers, it's about the people providing the care that will get you the numbers! The key to success is creating a work environment where caregivers feel empowered and motivated to help the organization be successful. While patient satisfaction is important, it is secondary to caregiver engagement.

Patient satisfaction scores are an indirect measurement of caregiver engagement.

This book was written to support and encourage the leaders who will face that challenge. It was written to help you celebrate those individuals who work tirelessly at the bedside every day. For this reason, I have used the term "caregiver" throughout the book, rather than "employees" or "staff members". These individuals are more than just an employee number; they are compassionate individuals who provide bedside care.

Help and support them during these difficult times, and in return, the bedside caregivers will want to do the same for you. They will strive to meet goals because they want to, not because they're told to do so. Don't get lost in the patient satisfaction scores and numbers. Instead, understand that if you care for the caregivers, they will provide the quality of care you are seeking, for the organization, and the patients and families that entrust their lives to them every day.

If the caregivers are happy, if they truly love what they're doing, then they'll want to be an energetic, supportive part of the process. Happiness breeds contentment, creating fulfilled caregivers, who feel motivated and empowered, to work toward a common goal, creating the ultimate patient experience. The scores and numbers will follow.

So, how do we do make our caregivers the focus of our efforts? It's not easy. The journey is long and requires patience, persistence, determination, and the occasional glass of wine. You need to rely on others and, at times, have faith that what you're asking for is actually getting accomplished. With struggle comes a heightened sense of excitement when reaching your final destination, which is a collaborative engaged team of high performers who want to provide patients with an experience that exceeds all expectations.

CHAPTER 1
DEVELOPING A GAME PLAN

SHOTS FIRED!

There are some situations in our careers and our lives that change us forever. Such an event occurred in my life at 5:30pm on September 29, when an off-duty police officer witnessed a woman trying to climb out of the passenger window of a moving car. As he got closer, he saw the driver yank her back into the car and punch her in the face.

He was an off-duty state trooper driving in his civilian car. He realized that the woman was in trouble, so he called ahead to the local police department and informed the dispatcher. Shortly thereafter, a uniformed officer approached the car and pulled the driver over to the side of the road. The driver was arrested without incident and brought to the hospital for bloodwork to rule out a possible DUI. As per protocol, a second officer was called and asked to assist the uniformed officer with the transport. That officer, who was off duty at the time of the call, grabbed his personal firearm rather than his service revolver and joined the uniformed officer in the emergency department.

The officer approached the caregiver in triage and asked if she could draw the driver's bloodwork, which was standard procedure in this case. She agreed, and the patient sat in the evaluation chair as the two officers stood guard. The bloodwork was drawn and paperwork was completed. It was at this time that the driver asked if he could use the bathroom before being transported to the local jail.

The caregiver pointed to where the bathroom was located and the plainclothes officer transported the patient to the bathroom, entering the room with him while the uniformed officer stood guard outside the door. Within seconds, things went wrong.

The emergency room technician, who had been speaking to the uniformed officer, reported seeing the bathroom door slowly open. Her attention turned to the bathroom, and she watched the plainclothes officer walk backward from the bathroom with his hands raised in the air. The emergency room technician then witnessed the barrel of a gun, held by the suspect, slowly appear from behind the bathroom door, pointed straight at the officer's chest.

"He's got his gun!" In a matter of seconds, chaos ensued. The uniformed officer looked up, and tried to pull his gun from his holster. Before he could remove it, the gunman turned the barrel toward him and fired 4 shots, striking the officer once in the abdomen and once in the head, a third bullet hit an emergency room technician in the neck as he attempted to flee, and the fourth bullet missed everyone and lodged in the wall just behind the 2 victims. The plainclothes officer then lunged at the shooter, trying to stop him. The shooter shoved him with his free hand and shot another bullet through his own extended hand, which stopped in the chest of the second officer.

After the shooting stopped, there was a deafening silence. The shooter then calmly walked over to the first officer, who had already sustained two gunshot wounds. He stood over him and, without compassion or sympathy, said, "Die, pig. Die." He fired his final bullet into his head execution style.

The shooter dropped the gun and exited the hospital through the emergency department waiting room. A unit clerk, angry at what had just happened, jumped over the desk, grabbed the gun, and chased after the shooter. The startled patients in the waiting room saw the shooter in a patient gown, bleeding, and being chased by a young man in blue scrubs (the unit clerk). Seeing a patient bleeding from the hand and running they assumed the unit clerk was the shooter, and as they placed calls from the waiting room to 911, they described the man with blue scrubs as the shooter possessing a gun.

The head of security heard the dispatcher state, "All-points bulletin. Shooter is in blue scrubs, tall white male." Wrong shooter! Thank goodness the security guard searched for and found the unit clerk, shouting, "Put the gun down or they're going to shoot you!" He put the gun down reluctantly, and thankfully, a second tragedy was avoided.

The actual shooter exited the emergency department and started running toward the park that surrounded the hospital, but then decided a better place to hide was the third floor of the parking garage. A tactical SWAT team arrived on the scene and started its search. Knowing that the suspect was injured, I quickly found the paramedic in charge of the scene. I pleaded with him to let me know when they found the shooter. Since he was bleeding, I knew he would need medical attention. "Please put him in the ambulance and drive to any hospital other than ours. This guy just tried to kill us." After 75 long minutes, they found the shooter hiding in the backseat of a car parked on the roof of the garage. Apparently, the blood trail from his wounded hand had led the SWAT team to him, and he was arrested without incident. As I listened to the police radio, I heard they had apprehended the suspect, and that they were escorting him down the back staircase to be treated by the trauma team. Despite my best efforts, we were now responsible for this person's well-being.

A True Test of What We Had Created

Regardless of my failed attempt to divert this individual, he now sat in the trauma room and the team had to treat him for his injuries. I remember asking myself, *How will they find the strength and courage to administer medical care for a person who just shot one of their own in the neck?* I entered the trauma room and excused all emergency room personnel who didn't need to be there. I gowned up, grabbed another nurse and, as two very large officers stood guard at the door with M-16 machine guns, we proceeded to take care of the patient. I recall that he was very calm as if nothing had even happened. There was no eye contact and not a word was spoken. We treated his hand wound, did an assessment for further injuries, and then quickly moved him to another area of the hospital to await surgery.

I remember being surprised at the emotions I felt immediately after he left the emergency department. Naturally, one would think my anger would get the best of me, and that it would then manifest into an emotional breakdown when the pressure of the situation was gone. Instead, I remember feeling an immense sense of pride. This team of caregivers, despite what was going on in their minds and in their hearts, focused on the job at hand, caring for those who needed them. A team of providers were assigned to each of the three shooting victims, another assigned to the shooter, and of course there were the countless others who were present prior to the chaos with medical issues that needed to be addressed.

After the shooter left the emergency department, I walked outside for a brief moment to collect my thoughts. My focus shifted from healing the physically wounded to supporting the emotionally scarred. Over 100 officers, 3 helicopters, and a mass of media trucks had converged onto our little community hospital. It was loud. It was chaotic. I walked back into the emergency department, and the first thing that hit me was the stark difference in energy. There were no screams, no crying. Instead, there was a calming silence. You could see the fear on their faces. You could feel the sadness seeping from their hearts. But there was still a job to be done and they were doing it. I will never forget that feeling. Through our tragedy came clarity. We were a team, there for each other, and bonded forever.

The Aftermath

After the tragedy, we made sure to provide support for everyone involved. This was clearly a tragic event. We held a critical stress debriefing that night and offered further psychiatric counseling. We told the caregivers, "You can take off for as long as you need so that you can recover mentally. We will provide you with resources and counseling. There is no rush to come back." After such an event, one would think that there would be someone who would take full advantage of that offer. Some took the offer of counseling, but not one person took longer than 3 days to return to work. The majority never missed a day.

In reality, we spend much of our lives with those we work with. As a leader, you put a plan in place, set the vision, and help everyone work toward it. We are often left asking, "Have we truly changed the culture yet? Is our vision a reality? Are we a team?" Through our tragedy came clarity, yes we were there for each other. The positive working culture that we had worked so hard to achieve was a reality. We were a team, and together we could accomplish anything, regardless of the circumstances.

HEALTHCARE IS A BUSINESS

Let's be very clear: like it or not, healthcare is a business. This is difficult to say as we like to believe that because we deal with life and death, emotions and cures, and human beings with their medical ailments, that there should be no price assigned to that experience. The truth is, however, that reimbursement of healthcare dollars has changed. The quality of the care you provide, and the cost at which you can provide it, plays a vital role in the success or failure of today's healthcare institutions.

The way people choose healthcare has changed as well. Healthcare choices used to be made with a patient's heart or brain, meaning that they chose hospitals in their community because it was where they were born or because it was their neighborhood hospital. Some chose healthcare services based on where their family physician admitted patients. I once had a person tell me they loved our hospital because our "cafeteria is the best." Yes, her choice was based on food preference! That is no longer the way healthcare is chosen. Instead of using one's brain or following one's heart, people now choose healthcare because of one deciding factor: their wallet.

Patients are deciding where they obtain their healthcare based on Affordable Care Act healthcare exchanges or private insurance companies' tiering systems. They're making these choices based on economics; they're looking for the most coverage for the least amount of money. Some have chosen plans with high deductibles and costly copays. Many are playing "medical roulette", selecting a minimal cost plan in the hopes that they never get sick and never need it.

The financial consideration continues when you look at how many people under the Affordable Care Act choose their healthcare coverage. Each person is asked to choose from programs offered in the exchanges. According to the Affordable Care Act fact page, there are nearly 49 million people around the country who were without access to healthcare coverage prior to the act's implementation[1]. Each exchange offers its customers a list of hospitals in their area and each of these hospitals are assigned a tier. The tier system is based on a hospital's quality scores and patient engagement ranking. For example, tier 1 hospitals have excellent quality scores as well as great patient engagement. Tier 2 hospitals have either average quality scores and good patient engagement or poor engagement and good quality scores. Finally, tier 3 hospitals have both poor quality and poor satisfaction scores[2].

These scores are important because the better the score, the lower the deductible that must be paid by the patient. For example, let's say a person decides to pick a tier 3 hospital because it's where her doctor sees patients

---

[1] Obamacare Facts. (2015, August 1). Retrieved August 1, 2015 from http://obamacarefacts.com/sign-ups/obamacare-enrollment-numbers/
[2] Affordable Care Act Update: Implementing Medicare Cost Savings. Retrieved March 15, 2015 from https://www.cms.gov/apps/docs/aca-update-implementing-medicare-costs-savings.pdf

or because it's located in her neighborhood. This decision was made with her heart. Unfortunately, with a tier 3 status, the hospital copay will be $2000. However, if she selects a tier 2 hospital, the copay would only be $1200. Even better, if the decision is to pick a tier 1 hospital, a hospital with great quality outcomes as well as a great patient experience ranking, the copay would only be $150. Even though her heart wants to go to the first hospital, her wallet is going to disagree[3].

This has been the federal government's answer to universal healthcare for those people who do not have insurance. Private insurance companies are now following the same philosophy. Their stance is why should we pay out more than what the government is paying? These private companies, however, have gone one step further. Private insurers have given healthcare institutions a mandate. If hospitals agree to accept Medicare rates, which would require them to drastically reduce costs (not easy to do immediately), then that insurer will label them as a tier 1 hospital. Tier 1 status is preferred by those that use the insurance, because the copays are much less than if they choose to go to a tier 3 hospital. Those hospitals that do not agree to accept Medicare rates can do so. They will receive more revenue per patient; however, they will also be listed as a tier 3 hospital, which has higher copays, forcing some current patients to seek healthcare at other institutions[4].

Private insurance companies will argue that this is not healthcare extortion, but, rather, it is a way to force healthcare institutions to decrease their costs. Their logic is that medical institutions could afford to accept Medicare rates if they lowered their costs, but unlike Medicare, the tiered system is based on acceptance of payment and not merit of the care provided.

Since hospitals will now be competing to gain patients, they must start to think differently. It is no longer solely about reputation, it is now about how much the patient can afford. We must accept business philosophies and determine how we can be better than "the other guy." Providing quality care is expected by the consumer. Businesses that are successful not only find ways to meet expectations, they strive to exceed them. Companies like

---

[3] Tiered Insurance Networks: Complicating Obamacare or Controlling Costs? Retrieved March 15, 2015 from http://www.cfah.org/blog/2014/tiered-insurance-networks-complicating-obamacare-or-controlling-costs
[4] Ibid

Disney, Chick-fil-A, and Southwest Airlines have all found ways to provide the positive experience you expect from businesses like theirs, and then give you even more. They set themselves apart from others by creating experiences that you would never have expected. If your hospital wants to compete for healthcare dollars, they too, must find a way to exceed the patient's expectations.

The Best Customer Experience

Finding ways to exceed people's expectations is what businesses try to do to stand out amongst the others. One of my favorite examples of exceeding expectations occurred as I walked through O'Hare International Airport. The expectation I'd had that day was that I should arrive an hour before my flight departed, wait to be seated on the plane, and then pray that I'd sit next to a normal person. On this one particular evening flight, as I walked to my gate, I saw that there was a large crowd cheering and laughing at the Southwest gate scheduled to fly to Atlanta. As I got closer to the gate, I became more intrigued by what was happening. In the middle of the seating area, just in front of the ticket counter, there was a Southwest employee who was handing miniature bean bags to those who were waiting to board. About 30 feet away was a wooden box with a hole cut in the middle. Each person with a bag stepped up to the line and tossed the bag at the hole. Curious, I asked another person watching this fun event why there were people playing a game in the middle of the airport. He told me that their flight to Atlanta had two available first class seats, but no one was willing to pay for the upgrade. So, Southwest was providing passengers with a chance to move up. The first person to throw the bag through the hole got the upgrade!

I didn't expect that, but boy, what a smart idea! This airline took a normal process, which we see every day in airports throughout the country, and made it fun. This airline found a way in that moment to exceed the expectation of the customers that support their business. That's why I love Southwest. They allow their employees the freedom to be creative and provide the best customer experience possible. Why does this happen? It happens because their employees are engaged and are empowered to do what is right for the customer. This is how healthcare must change its thinking. It's not only about diagnoses, treatment, and medication anymore, it's about finding ways to make your business stand out from the rest. It's about discovering ways to exceed a patient and their families' expectations.

If you do the unexpected, it will be noticed.

So, how do we come up with programs that are new and creative in healthcare? It's not easy, but it can be done. There are, of course, basic business principles that must be followed. New programs that are created must be financially prudent, adding value without adding costs. For example, one day in the emergency department, I pulled our Best Practice Committee together and informed them, "Hey, guys, we're going to do something today, and I know it's going to be a hit!" That always generates some cautious interest!

Their response was, "Oh no, not again!"

I continued by saying, "Today, when people come in on this hot summer day, we're going to offer them and their families a cool wet towel for their faces while they wait. I want us to say, "Welcome to the emergency department. How can I help you?" After our patients tell us their reason for their visit, we'll reply, "You may have to wait a few minutes. We apologize. In order to make your wait a bit more comfortable, may I offer you a cool towel for your face?"

What do you think my staff thought when I told them this? What are you thinking right now? They thought it was unnecessary, crazy, and just more work for them. I reminded them our patients are anxious individuals with medical problems who have chosen us for their healthcare needs on this very hot day. This would certainly exceed what they were expecting when they walked in the door, and it would add nothing more to our day than offering a cool towel to a stressed-out patient. The next question I answered was, "What if they don't want the towel?" I replied that the offer would then at least be acknowledged and hopefully appreciated. It was certainly not expected.

Think about it. When a patient comes to the hospital or the emergency department, they expect to see a doctor, they expect to be correctly diagnosed, and they expect to get some treatment or medication to help them feel better. That's what they expect and that's usually what they receive. But what if they receive just a little something extra? What if we were able, even by some seemingly small gesture, to provide patients with something that they didn't expect? If we do that, we've made an impact.

If we want people to choose us, we must find a way to truly transform the patient experience. We need to find those things that will make that patient's experience just a little better—something that will go beyond what's simply expected.

Our future depends on our ability to think differently. What happens in business when you fail to reinvent your business? You'll lose your customer base, and without a customer base, you lose money, and without revenue you will eventually go out of business. The future of healthcare is uncertain. It is difficult to imagine vacant hospitals with "out of business" signs posted in the windows. And yet, if we cannot adapt from a clinically-focused care environment to one with a business focus, then there will be some hospitals that will close their doors forever.

The closure of hospitals is a real threat to the future of healthcare. In an article by the *Huffington Post* titled "Hospitals Facing More Credit Downgrades, Threat of Closure Looms", they acknowledge that hospitals are struggling to get the cash they need in order to remain profitable. Their credit scores are being downgraded, making it difficult to borrow cash. Like any other business, hospitals rely on credit scores to borrow money. Lower credit scores equal higher interest rates and the chance that borrowing money will not be possible.[5] In addition, if insurance continues to redirect patients to lower-cost outpatient care, like urgent care and ambulatory care centers, then acute care hospitals will have to find new ways to provide care in order to remain profitable. Healthcare has changed. We need to make sure we adapt to that change.

What the New Healthcare Means to You

The changes occurring in healthcare today are the most challenging since Lyndon B. Johnson signed the Medicare Act in 1965. Not since then have healthcare institutions been forced to look at every aspect of their business in the interest of financial survival. It seems like each day, there is a new metric that needs to be reported or a government regulation that adds yet another task to the already overworked bedside caregiver. Revenues are shrinking, and the workforce needs to be reduced in order to meet the financial shortcomings[6].

This model is unsustainable. How do we provide the same level of

---

[5] The Huffington Post (2012, April 7). Retrieved July 20, 2015 from http://www.huffingtonpost.com/2012/04/17/hospital-credit-downgrade_n_1431582.html

[6] As Medicare and Medicaid Turn 50, Use of Private Health Plans Surges. Retrieved August 7, 2015 from http://www.nytimes.com/2015/07/30/us/as-medicare-and-medicaid-turn-50-use-of-private-health-plans-surges.html

quality care for the patient and their families with a workforce that has been reduced due to a budget crisis or operations improvement strategy? The regulatory requirements are the same. The public expectation of quality compassionate care is the same. The expectations from senior administration are the same. So, as a leader, how do you get your overworked and overwhelmed bedside caregivers to want to work their hardest to create the best patient experience possible? It is not easy. The uncertain future brings anxiety, which, in turn, is transferred through the caregivers to the patient. You will never get the patient satisfaction scores you are looking for without happy caregivers. Would you be willing to go the extra mile to create an excellent patient experience that exceeds the expectation for an organization who doesn't value you or your opinions? Would you be willing to think outside the box and find creative solutions to problems if you felt that your boss didn't respect you? It starts with leadership. Each of us is expected to be a leader, whether it is as a bedside caregiver providing an excellent patient experience or as a leader helping the bedside caregiver do their job. Both are required if you want to create the ultimate experience for both patients and the people who are caring for them.

LEADERSHIP

My Journey to Leadership

My early nursing career began with a variety of experiences. I started my career as a telemetry nurse essentially because no one would hire me as a new nurse in the emergency department. After 11 very long months, I was finally hired as a nurse in the emergency department. I worked in the inner city where the patients manipulated the healthcare system in many ways in order to fulfill their other needs, looking for meals to satisfy their hunger, or a place to sleep for the night. They did so by making up illnesses or injuries. I realize to the layperson this may sound cynical and harsh, but if you've worked in this type of environment, you're well aware of what I mean. When I was ready to move on, I left to try my hand at travel nursing and then decided to hone my clinical skills as a flight nurse, a job I had aspired to since the beginning of my career and one that I loved. However, life changed, and the time came to start a family.

I returned home. Uncertain of what I wanted to do, I reached out to my mentor and former nurse manager, Fern Gordon, with whom I'd maintained a relationship during the years I'd been away. No matter where I resided, I would come back once a year—the day after Christmas—and we would get together for lunch. I told Fern I didn't know what my next step in nursing would be. She looked at me and asked, "Have you ever thought about leadership?" To be honest, I had not. I didn't think that leadership was for me. I didn't want to have to go to work 5 days a week, 8 hours a day. I wanted to do my three 12-hour shifts, focus on the clinical, and then go home.

She told me about a leadership position where she worked—she was recently promoted to nursing director—and she wanted me to help her "turn around the emergency department" as her nurse manager. She told me that it was a great place to work. It was a little hospital nestled in the suburbs and surrounded by woods and wildlife. After some careful thought, I decided to take on this new challenge.

I quickly learned that the challenge was going to be greater than I had imagined.

During my first day on the job, I discovered that the group that I was leading had had 4 managers over the last 5 years. The unit had a reputation for unfriendly staff and poor care.

I remember thinking, *Do I really want to put myself through this?* But I've never backed away from difficult things, and I wasn't about to start now. I wanted to take on the impossible and, where others had failed, succeed. That's what leadership is about. It's about finding new ways to do old, outdated things. It's about taking on challenges that will test your will at times and provide you with goal-exceeding excitement at other times. It's an opportunity to bring a group of individuals together and to help them work as a team to provide compassionate care to people on their worst day.

Many things are involved in the making of a leader. There are those who are born natural leaders, while there are others that need to be nurtured. This process takes time and requires many things. Our life experiences and the people we meet along our life's journey shape who we are as leaders. We adopt the traits of those we admire, and we avoid the behaviors of those we do not like. When I took on that first leadership role, I didn't suddenly become a leader. In many ways, I had been developing as a leader for many years. I'm still developing today with every experience, every success, and more importantly, every failure.

The Desire to Lead

I believe that for most people, the initial desire to be a leader is within them. You see it on the sports fields or in the classrooms every day. There are children on sports teams who tell the other kids to keep their heads high after a loss or encourage a teammate the loudest when they are up to bat. There are those children who are first to volunteer to read to the group and others who offer to help other students when they're struggling in class.

One of my first influences was my elementary school teacher, Mr. Strong. When I was in the 5th grade, I wanted to be on the safety patrol. Mr. Strong was the teacher in charge. I can vividly remember the day he made me a lieutenant. I remember thinking that 5th graders aren't allowed to be lieutenants; that privilege is usually reserved for 6th graders. For whatever reason, he gave me that rank, which only encouraged me to prove I could do it. And I did. Mr. Strong promoted me to captain the following year. I often wonder why he made that choice. Did he see something in me? Did he know how his decision would help me to form some of my leadership abilities as a kid and the effect that would have later in my life?

This happens with all of us. We learn from those around us and we pick up the traits that we view as positive and learn to overcome or minimize the traits that we view as negative. We observe, learn, and shape ourselves for the future.

Create Some Followers

There are things we can do to improve ourselves as leaders. Each person who takes on a leadership role will have their strengths and of course their weaknesses. There is, however, one thing we all need in order to succeed as a leader: willing followers. Tom Atchison, the author of *Followership: A Practical Guide to Aligning Leaders and Followers* predicates being a good leader on the basic premise, "Without followers there are no leaders."[7] I love this philosophy, and it is a fundamental concept that all new leaders who are working to understand the importance of engaging the caregivers should understand. You may think you're a leader, but, if you look behind you and nobody's following, you're nothing more than a task manager.

So, how do you build those relationships and get people to trust you?

---

[7] Atchison, T. (2004). *Followership: A Practical Guide to Aligning Leaders and Followers.* Chicago, Il: Heath Administration Press

We will discuss the steps required to achieve followers in later chapters, but before that process starts, you must first examine your own individual behavior. It's a great leader who understands that they must set the example for others to follow. Define for caregivers what behaviors are expected, and show that you are willing to be the first to exhibit them.

For example, a skill I knew I needed to improve upon was being a good listener. "Just listen to them," was a common phrase that Fern would repeat to me. Block out your thoughts and jaded opinions and *listen*. I admit this was incredibly difficult for me in the beginning. Most people who are in leadership are thinkers; they are ambitious individuals who have lots of ideas and plans. And our first instinct is to implement it all! Most caregivers will tell you that what is important to them is they want to be heard. It is impossible to overdo listening. When I started as the manager of the emergency department, I came in on nights. I came in on weekends. I simply came in to meet with caregivers and to listen to their ideas and concerns. After all, who knows the system better than those working at the bedside every day?

I started each meeting with the same purposeful questions:

- What can I do to make your job better?
- What can I do to help remove the roadblocks to delivering the best care possible?

All of our conversations would be centered around what I referred to as "creating the ultimate working experience." This experience creates an environment where you come into work every day and say, "I really love what I do!"

When I first started my leadership journey, I was so excited. My enthusiasm and eagerness to get started was bubbling out through my pores. So many of the issues that were presented to me were easy fixes. I wanted to make an impression and show every caregiver that I was here to help. I started making changes, lots of changes. It was exciting. However, making changes that would make the unit better did not improve the morale; instead, it made it worse. Even those who wanted the change felt overwhelmed. I was confused, and, to tell you the truth, a bit disappointed that my efforts were not appreciated. It all became apparent to me when Fern, my director, came to me and said, "We need to talk."

I followed her to her office and took a seat. She asked, "Charles, tell me what you're doing." I outlined the plan, giving her my ideas, thoughts, and processes for making change. She took it all in, listened, and said, "It's too much too fast. You're trying to change everything at once without understanding the dynamics of change. People need to feel comfortable with change. I know it's needed, but you can't do it all at once. They'll be so overwhelmed, they'll miss the great things that you're trying to do. Just take it all in for six months. Remember to just *Listen* and write down your ideas; be patient, but do nothing."

I needed to understand both how to motivate the group and each individual, and then use that knowledge to enlist the caregivers to make the needed change. I needed to relinquish control and believe those who worked for me would want to work in a place that works for them.

So, that's what I did. I backed off for 6 months. I think the restraint gave me a hernia. Telling a guy with ADD to do nothing is like telling a diabetic working in a candy factory they can't sample any of the product. The takeaway here is that it was a good leadership lesson. You can't change everything at once. You have to be patient. Being patient and listening will help foster caregiver engagement and caregiver engagement is the key to being successful.

WHERE DO I START?

This is perhaps the most frequent question I am asked. They want to make a change. They want to get the results but the process to get there seems overwhelming. One step at a time! A new leader or a seasoned veteran, it makes no difference; we all have to start at the same point, identifying where opportunities exist for success. Once the opportunities are identified then the plan can begin to take shape.

This book is designed to structure this process. As each chapter unfolds, you will see the chronological steps that are required to engage staff and begin to transform the patient experience.

Game Plan Tip: Developing the Game Plan

The question I get asked most often by leaders who reach out for help is: "Where do I start?" I answer them with the same answer each time: "Relax, take a deep breath, and ask yourself the three game plan questions."

1.   Why do we need this change?

Start by asking yourself why the change is needed. Are there widespread problems, or isolated incidents? Is this a product of hospital policies and processes, or is this an issue with meshing team personalities? Slow down and start gathering the facts. This first question centers you and helps you to feel positive that there is about to be a plan.

2.   What information do I need to start to make change?

You may feel that you know what the problems are, but this opinion may be one-sided. Ask the staff. Understand their frustrations. Where are their roadblocks? Have town hall meetings and collect information. Do this for all shifts. Include everyone in on the conversation: nurses, assistants, unit clerks, and yes, even the physicians. Write it down. Don't interrupt. Don't try to fix it. Just listen.

3.   What resources do I have to help me plan?

If you have a leadership team, are they all on the same page? Has nursing administration been made aware of your plan? Do they support it? If not, what do you and your team need to do to educate them? Are there outside resources who can help if needed?

Culture change is difficult. It didn't get this bad overnight, so why would you think it will get better any faster? Take it step by step, find caregivers who are excited to be a part of the change, and be consistently patient. Before you know it, staff engagement will occur, and the patient's experience will be transformed.

CHAPTER 2
CREATING A SENSE OF EXCITEMENT

LET THE JOURNEY BEGIN

How many times have you shown up for your shift, looked at who was working, and said, "This is going to be a good day"? Have you ever found yourself looking at the people you'd be working with during your shift and suddenly start to get a migraine? All caregivers have experienced these fluctuations in feelings during their careers. I'm sure we would all agree that if we could create the ultimate working experience, then we would choose to work with the people in the former group, and not the latter. Creating a working environment like this takes time, but it can be done.

The first step to success is to first acknowledge the stress that accompanies any kind of change. Especially when you're trying to change a negative culture that has been present in the workplace for a very long time.

Change is a Very Bad Word

Before you can make change, you need to understand it. The greatest challenge for any leader is leading people through change. Unfortunately, many organizations are facing their toughest challenges in decades. From a caregiver perspective, these challenges have done nothing more than place more and more responsibility on them. The burden of healthcare requirements and regulations are falling on the backs of those who practice at the bedside. They are overworked and overwhelmed, "So please don't give me anything more to do!" That's how they see it. More regulations and more metrics equals more stress and more work.

When we start on the journey of change, we need to understand that patience is one of the most important skills we can have as leaders. Why? Because change doesn't happen quickly. The policy or process may change, but the culture and work environment around it will take time. There will be setbacks along the way. We'll move forward, we'll make progress, and then we'll lose ground. There will be times of regression. There will be times of challenge. It can be a very stressful time.

I speak from experience. After accepting a leadership role, I found myself overwhelmed and frustrated. It affected my personality, personal life, and eventually my health. After the first 12 months in the role of leader, stressed by all the changes that needed to occur, I found myself lying on a table, having a cardiac catheterization because of the persistent chest pains I had experienced at the ripe old age of 33. The caregivers were trying to kill me! I was trying to initiate change! The pressure, the constant sabotage, the constant questioning, and the constant regression was sometimes too much to bear.

I remember saying to myself, *You have to have confidence in the vision. Stick to the plan!* Change is a slow process. Understand that fact, accept it, and success is then possible.

Change is Uncomfortable

As the process of change begins, leaders must understand that when it comes to effecting change in a department, or an organization, it's uncomfortable for some people. It's anxiety producing for others. Bottom line is that some, if not most, don't like it! When leaders point out a group's shortcomings and say, "You need to do this differently," often the first reaction from that group is to fight the change and hang onto the way they've always done it. They may feel that, "This is my system; this is my process; this is my routine." You're attempting to force them out of that comfortable routine toward some unknown. That's uncomfortable. That takes effort. And effort is energy.

There are many forces that suck the energy from those working in healthcare. Caregivers are already expending so much energy just dealing with the day-to-day demands of their jobs—the day-to-day demands of the patients they care for, the providers and colleagues they interact with, and the families they try to support. It's not easy.

So, how can leaders initiate change that helps the caregivers accept the plan? In other words, how do you turn your ideas into our ideas? The first thing that you must understand is that change is difficult. Accepting that reality is the first step a leader can make in order to have an empathetic understanding of the caregivers struggle with the change. Dr. John Kotter states in his book *Leading Change* (2012, pg. 4), "...the downside of change is inevitable. Whenever human communities are forced to adjust to shifting conditions, pain is ever present."[8] Understanding the stress the change will cause, and acknowledging it, will help to form the necessary bond to help the change process be successful.

I think there are some other things leaders can understand about change that can help to nurture the caregivers to accept it. Based on my experience, the second most important thing that a leader can understand is the more you include the caregivers in the decision, the greater the buy in you will experience. If caregivers are forced to change they will resist. However, if they are given the ability to control that change, they're more likely to accept it.

A great example of this occurred in the beginning of my leadership career when it was voiced loudly that one of the biggest complaints was the schedule. Some people got what they wanted, while others did not. Weekend shifts were not evenly distributed. Some people had to do 3 different shifts in 1 week. The bottom line is that they didn't think the schedule was fair. A change was needed, but how should I change the process? The answer was that I should not be changing the process, *they* should! So, after giving them some guidelines, we turned the decision over to the caregivers. They worked it out amongst themselves and came up with a plan that worked for most people. Those who did not agree with the new process had to discuss their issues with the scheduling committee and explain to their peers, not me, why they didn't like it. Accountability and ownership were all on the caregivers, and because of this, the change had greater acceptance.

If someone from administration starts off a meeting by saying, "This is how we're changing things," people are less likely to respond favorably. Why? Because it wasn't their idea. They didn't have any input. They're just being told what to do. People react more favorably to change when they understand it, when they can see how the change will benefit them and, especially when they've had some part to play in designing the change.

---

[8] Kotter, J. (2012). *Leading Change* (1st ed.). Boston, MA: Harvard Business School Press.

To ease the anxiety, we trial all applicable changes for 30 days. Even if we try something and after 7 days, caregivers are saying, "We hate this," we keep it going for another 23 days. We want to ensure that the uncomfortable feeling the caregivers are having isn't just related to being uncomfortable with change and we can't determine that after one week. So, we ride it out for 30 days to ensure that it's the actual process that isn't working.

Nothing About Me, Without Me

The thing about change is that although the caregivers generally do not respond favorably to change and would probably say that they don't "like" it, it's really all about degrees. In fact, there are rules in leadership that help you determine the amount of resistance that you might encounter when you are trying to bring about change. For example, change is much easier when the person being impacted can control the process to some degree. When they have a say in that decision then they will likely buy into and adopt the change concept.[9] Despite your best efforts, there will always be a nervous energy present. Understand and accept it, then find a way to use it.

This feeling of uneasiness occurred for my staff every year in October. This was the month that I left to attend the Emergency Nurses Association Leadership Conference. When I'd tell my staff where I was going, they'd say, "Is it that time already?" They knew what was coming. They knew that I would return from the conference with a brain full of new ideas and programs that I would want to try. To me, those new ideas represented possibilities. To my staff, they represented change.

The National Patient Safety Foundations Executive Summary (2003) used the phrase "Nothing about me, without me" when identifying the direct causal relationship between the inclusion of patients into their daily care, like medications and treatment courses, and the positive affects it has on compliance and healing.[10] Employees, like patients, want, and need, to

---

[9] 8 Tips to Help Managers and Employees Deal With Organizational Change. (2010). Retrieved May 10, 2015 from http://www.peterstark.com/managers-employees-organizational-change.

[10] National Patient Safety Foundation & Patient and Family Advisory Council (2000). National agenda for action: Patients and families in patient safety; Nothing about me, without me. Retrieved August 26, 2015 from http://c.ymcdn.com/sites/www.npsf.org/resource/collection/ABAB3CA8-4E0A-41C5-A480-6DE8B793536C/Nothing_About_Me.pdf

be participants in the change process. The focus of leaders should first be to involve the staff in the change process if success is the desired end result.

Administration uses terms like "metrics" and "target goals", but caregivers only hear, "work, work and then more work." Stop chasing the numbers! If you chase the numbers, caregivers will feel that it is not about the care they provide, it is about meeting a number set by someone who has no idea what they do. So find a way to make it theirs and give them control of the change in order to secure the engagement needed to be successful.

Change Takes Time

Even with their support change will take time. When I first started as a leader, I was challenged. We had a 45 percent vacancy rate and our turnover rate was over 50 percent. Those are staggering numbers. I needed time to turn those numbers around. We didn't get to that place in 3 months, so I needed to understand that it wasn't getting better in 3 months. And in fact, as often happens with change, things might get even worse before they get better.

Over time, I had to have faith in the vision we set. I believed that if we stood our ground, if we focused on the right things—the things that were important to our hospital, to the department, and to the staff—that at the end of 3 years, we would achieve our goal. My hope was instead of talking about vacancy rates, the conversation would be about how to manage the waiting list of people wanting to come to work in our department. That was the vision, and I needed to keep everyone focused on it.

Sustaining Change

To be effective, we must sustain change so that it can be embedded within the culture. Either the change is aligned with the current culture or, if it is not, then the long process of changing the culture must begin. Strong culture drives strong results, starting with engaged caregivers.

Perhaps the most important thing when it comes to change is taking time to remember the past. Before you look to the future, you must examine the past and learn from it. What other programs has the staff lived through? What was the most recent program? Why did it fail? Are there still parts of that system that exist today? If there have been too many of those "flavor of the week" initiatives in your organization, it's not surprising that caregivers may be resistant, thinking this is just another waste of their time. They've become cynical. They don't think it'll work because they've seen it before, and they think it's just "one of those programs."

An organization that understands the importance of culture is Chick-fil-A. According to their website, Chick-fil-A was founded in 1946 and is a privately-held company that operates according to the faith-based principles of its founder, Truett Cathy.[11] These principles can be somewhat polarizing to some, but based on my experience, the company is always trying to find ways to exceed the expectation of its customer. During my workshops, I will ask the audience to name a company that always goes above and beyond for their customers. To my amazement, no matter where I am in this country, the same three companies are usually shouted out immediately. On almost every occasion, Chick-fil-A is one of those three.

Why? One of the things that makes Chick-fil-A stand out is their customer service. No matter what Chick-fil-A you walk into, you are always greeted with the same response, "It's my pleasure." Not: "No problem." Not: "Okay." Not an unintelligible grunt. But rather, "It's my pleasure." That leaves an impression. This is fast food they're selling. The Ritz-Carlton has the same greeting, but they're a luxury hotel. Chick-fil-A is selling fast food. Do you know how hard it is to get a teenage workforce to all say, "It's my pleasure?" It's just one of the things that helps them stand out amongst the other fast food chains.

What else do they do to exceed expectations? The response I often receive from my audiences includes, "They don't stand behind the counter—servers are out on the floor, providing table service." No checking Facebook or the latest upload to Instagram. They are productive and give the customer something that exceeds their expectation. This is fast food, people! I always like to wonder what that leadership meeting was like when the owner said, "We are going to do table service at all of our restaurants." I'm sure someone was at that meeting and said to themselves, "No one does table service at fast food restaurants." Exactly. No one does it, and that's why we are going to be the first.

It doesn't take much to exceed an expectation. So often we get tied up in the big programs that cost lots of money and rely on multiple resources for the benefit of the patient experience. It is about finding a way to stand out and be different than your competitors. Healthcare needs to change its thinking.

---

[11] Chick-fil-A. (2014). Company fact sheet. Retrieved July 6, 2015 from http://www.chick-fil-a.com/Company/Highlights-Fact-Sheets

We need to learn from successful businesses. I will say it again, healthcare is now a business. Think about it, the care you provide is now evaluated and rated on the internet. Our entire business entity is now ranked like other businesses, such as hotels on trip advisor or that toaster on Amazon. The 5-star rating system is now used to evaluate each hospital. Patients, or should we say customers (please don't call them customers, I'm just trying to make a point), do their research before picking a healthcare provider. We need to win their business. The only way to do that is to exceed their expectations and provide them with a service that they would never expect.

This book's main focus is not about the business plan to achieve this transformation, it is about engaging the caregivers so that they *want* to provide the kind of compassionate care that exceeds our patients' expectations. My hope is that the following chapters provide you with a road map for success and the knowledge needed to develop a culture that is based on accountability, motivation, and teamwork.

I can promise you one thing, when your culture changes and you can see and feel the motivation and engagement start to take hold, you will be amazed at what a team of highly motivated, compassionate team members can do to create the ultimate healing and working environment.

My Personal Leadership Journey

I knew that the changes that needed to be made, to engage the caregivers that I was now responsible for, would be a challenge. Engaging and motivating the bedside caregiver takes time, and time was something I didn't think I had. This was the feeling I remember having when I accepted my first opportunity to lead an emergency department. I wasn't sure I could be a good leader, but my mentor saw potential. I had so many ideas I wanted to implement. There was so much I wanted to fix or tweak. There were caregivers who were superstars, while there were others who just needed to go. I spent long hours at work developing a plan to make the changes I felt were needed. But before I could get started there was one fundamental concept that I needed to understand…*No one likes change.*

Changing culture is the most difficult thing to do in leadership. It is even more difficult to define the actual process that it takes to make that change. I use a simple formula for success. No research. No focus groups. Just years of experience helping poor performing units pull together as a team and achieve wonderful results. Complicated plans can be frustrating to follow and the possibility of success decreases quickly. Don't overthink it, and keep the end result as the main focus. If you learn how to motivate your team and empower them to make the changes necessary to create their own version of what the ultimate working experience looks like, then true caregiver engagement will occur. This is demonstrated by the following formula, which will be the backbone of everything that we discuss from this point on.

Motivation × Empowerment = Caregiver Engagement

Caregivers must be motivated. They need to feel that there's a purpose to their work, and the end result must be worth the difficult process necessary to achieve it. Let's admit it. Healthcare is getting more difficult. With less resources and increased regulation, it is difficult to provide the experience we want for all of our patients. It is also challenging to motivate a multigenerational workforce that is overwhelmed and overworked.

Empowerment must be paired with motivation. Feeling a sense of worth and belonging is essential in motivating a workforce. So what is true empowerment? I like to ask leaders to describe how they empower the bedside caregiver. So many times, they say that they empower staff by giving them tasks to complete. This type of thinking is common in healthcare leadership, but this practice is not empowerment. It is an opportunity to strategize how best to complete an already decided upon task. No creative thought processes are involved.

Caregiver engagement is manifested when the caregivers are given the freedom to explore different ways to meet goals and find solutions to problems affecting the department without oversight from leadership. That trust must be developed between caregiver and leader. This can be a struggle for both groups. However, if it can be achieved, staff will be more likely to feel empowered to find solutions to problems instead of simply complaining about the issues that affect them.

There are common leader failures when trying to develop this level of trust. I know of leaders who try to empower staff but when there is the slightest delay in correcting the problem they take over and say, "Okay, you tried it your way, now we're going to do it my way." Allowing your bedside caregivers the freedom to try something and fail, learn from that failure, and then create a new way to meet the goal provides them with an opportunity to make a change and be accountable to it. If they have a say in the vision, culture, and decisions of the department that directly affect their work lives, then they are more likely to work to resolve issues or follow their own decisions.

MOTIVATIONAL THEORY

Hierarchy of Needs

Maslow's Hierarchy of Needs

When considering motivation from a healthcare perspective, I always seem to return to Abraham Maslow. I have studied many motivational theorists; however, I believe Maslow provides a framework for understanding motivation in the workplace. He framed his model in the form of a hierarchy, now called "Maslow's hierarchy," and proposed that there was a process that humans moved through beginning with physiological needs (basic) and ending with self-actualization (high level).[12]

Healthcare leaders can determine motivational triggers using this hierarchy of needs so that they can help caregivers perform at their highest level. For example, exhaustion and the need for rest may motivate a caregiver to sleep. If caregivers are hungry and suffering from lack of sleep, their focus is likely to be on their hunger and tiredness, not on the patient's needs. A desire for belonging may lead caregivers to exhibit certain behaviors to become more likeable or lovable. And if they're afraid, it's unlikely they're ready to engage in productive and positive relationships in the workplace.

This isn't an entirely linear process, though. Caregivers move up and down the hierarchy frequently. As leaders, the goal is to ensure caregivers' basic (physiological and safety) needs are met so they can engage in productive workplace relationships, feel good about what they do, and become fully engaged, contributing members of their own department. It's a lofty goal, but one that can be attained.

The Nurse's Hierarchy of Needs

The needs discussed by Maslow are realized over an extended period of time. Self-actualization may occur over a few days, few months, or few years, while some individuals never discover their own potential. As leaders,

---

[12] Maslow's Hierarchy of Needs. Retrieved February 24, 2015 from http://www.edpsycinteractive.org/topics/conation/maslow.html.

we sometimes focus too much on the future and neglect the caregiver's present needs. What is going to make caregivers happy now or in the next 5 minutes? What will make the caregivers' day better over the course of the next 12-hour shift that we can try to make happen so they feel valued and respected? Understanding this can help caregivers see you as a person who understands their needs. Leadership is not a daily thing; it is an every minute thing.

I believe nurses have a unique hierarchy of needs as they're working 12-hour shifts. If leaders understand this they can help use it as a beginning step to motivate caregivers and ultimately create followers. In the Figure 2-1, I have simplified Maslow's theory to illustrate what I believe caregivers most desire in a 12-hour shift.

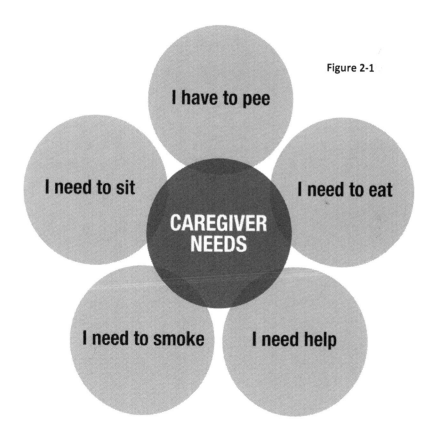

Figure 2-1

I have to pee

I need to sit

I need to eat

CAREGIVER NEEDS

I need to smoke

I need help

When I was a staff nurse, I remember thinking to myself, "I don't think I peed today." It wasn't until I got back home to my front door and started the "gotta go" dance that it actually sunk in.

Most caregivers are concerned about their breaks, schedule, food, and bodily functions during their shift. It is more important to the caregiver to meet each need as the day unfolds. It's a good place to start building quality working relationships.

Focusing on the immediate shift needs for caregivers is a quick way to help leaders to build relationships that are based on mutual respect. This is an immediate action that any leader can do for their staff. Later in the book, we will discuss other results-proven strategies for creating and maintaining such relationships.

Intrinsic and Extrinsic Motivation

Positive Intrinsic Motivation

Intrinsic motivation is, simply put, motivation from within. It's our own internal drive to do something. It is a desire driven by an innate sense of self-worth rather than by any external reward. Richard Ryan and Edward Deci (2000) postulated three innate psychological needs—competence, autonomy, and relatedness—"which yield enhanced self-motivation and mental health when satisfied and lead to diminished motivation and well-being when thwarted."[13] For instance, we may be intrinsically motivated to take a class in photography, learn scuba diving or yoga, or to develop a new language skill because we've always wanted to learn that skill and the idea of learning a new language is personally exciting. An intrinsic desire motivates an individual to acquire a skill, complete a task, or work toward a goal.

It is absolutely imperative to understand and recognize the driving motivational factors and acknowledging them when the opportunity presents itself. Intrinsic motivation can be realized as competence, autonomy, relatedness, and meaningful purpose.

Competence is our ability to apply our skills and training to our best abilities and have pride (or be motivated) by a job well done. As leaders, we want to provide bedside caregivers with the best chance to succeed. Finding the strengths of each caregiver is important. Doing a task that you are good at leads to success, which, in turn, self-motivates that individual to seek out other opportunities that have the potential to provide those same feelings. Our challenge as leaders is to determine what motivates each individual and

---

[13] Ryan, R.M., & Deci, E.L. (2000). Self-Determination Theory and the Facilitation of Intrinsic Motivation, Social Development, and Well-Being. American Psychologists, 55(1), 68-78.

use that to get the most out of each caregiver. The opportunity to realize our potential provides a sense of satisfaction and motivation to continue to meet the goals of that team or individual. Whether that be completing an assigned task or supporting the vision and culture of the department.

I remember the first time I was assigned the charge nurse role. I felt really good about myself. Why? Because somebody had enough faith in me to say, "I believe in your ability to run this unit while I'm not here. I trust you." That assigned task inspired me to do the best job possible but more importantly, my confidence was boosted when I was able to competently complete the task that was assigned to me. I remember loving that feeling and then urging my boss to give me more opportunities to lead others.

High-performing organizations and leaders understand the importance of this motivational concept. They identify what each individual's talents are and capitalize on utilizing those skills to build confidence within each caregiver. When a caregiver is successful at completing a task or accomplishing a goal, they then become motivated to do more.

Autonomy can occur any time caregivers work independently and control their own working environment. In such situations, they are more likely to be motivated to ensure that environment is the best possible. Over the course of your career, you will undoubtedly work for a leader who is considered to be a "micromanager". This type of leader must be involved in all decisions and have some control over everything that occurs within the department. Although self-satisfying for that leader, caregiver engagement will be lost when they realize that there is no autonomy in the work place. When caregivers are allowed to express their opinions, create solutions for their department's problems and can practice independently (while maintaining the fundamental focus that all decisions should be based on "Is this the right thing to do for the patients or my fellow teammates?") then they will be empowered to do so. This sense of autonomy brings a sense of pride, which intrinsically motivates an individual to search out more opportunities that will provide this kind of positive feeling.

Relatedness is when each of us strives to create and maintain healthy relationships with our fellow team members. The bond creates a sense of belonging and in that bonding relationship people are motivated to help and support each other. The relationship between caregivers and leaders is no different. Staff members want to know that leaders have an empathetic understanding about who they are and what they do. It is very unlikely that someone will "go the extra mile" for someone they do not respect.

The more relatedness that occurs, the more understanding can be realized. How do you relate to staff if you are the one in charge of holding them accountable? Listen to them, support them, and make them a prominent factor when it comes to the decisions that affect their working environment. You can even be their friend. Yes, their friend. I hear all the time that leaders cannot be friends with the caregivers who work for them, that it blurs the line of authority. I disagree. Can you hang out at a local drinking establishment and take turns being the designated driver? No. Respect is still required. However, I believe the bedside caregivers want to know that you're human, that you're as fallible as they are, and that you're willing to admit it. The more real, the more human, you can be, the more likely they're going to relate to you.

Meaningful purpose is what I believe is a fourth motivating factor, which perhaps resonates as the most humanistic. This motivating factor comes when a task or job provides an inner sense of accomplishment, or fulfills a personal belief, which then gives a sense of pride and belonging. Individuals who are motivated by a sense of meaningful purpose continue to seek out opportunities that help foster this feeling. For example, when a person volunteers at a local homeless shelter because they empathize with people who suffer from mental illness, they feel a sense of meaningful purpose because they are helping to support those who are affected. This feeling produces a positive outcome for the homeless and those who are helping, as well as the individual who is motivated by the positive feelings of their own personal act. When staff feel that their opinions matter, that their ideas are considered, and their comments are taken seriously, they will make choices aligned with the department or organization's goals, but consistent with their own needs for meaningful purpose.

Healthcare is a team sport, no doubt about it. We rely on our fellow team members to work together to provide the best care possible. As individuals, bedside caregivers must find a way to survive in a hectic and stressful healthcare environment, and leaders must find a way to support their efforts and motivate them to do more. With less resources, increasing regulatory responsibilities, and an aging patient population, who present with more diverse and complicated health concerns, it is imperative to maintain caregiver morale. This can be done by providing work that is meaningful, can relate to an individual, and provide a sense of pride when a task is done or a culture is changed.

Negative Intrinsic Motivation

Negative intrinsic motivation presents itself in various and sometimes escalating forms. For example, graduate nurses are sometimes negatively motivated to do well during their orientation. After graduating school, they enter the work place and it is that fear of failure that motivates an individual to work hard to ensure that they successfully complete orientation. Perhaps it's a lack of confidence that motivates them to seek out additional information after their shift is over. I know for some nurses (myself included), it's hard to think back to the day that we first walked onto a nursing unit. The feeling that sat in the pit of your stomach and the chant that you would mentally say over and over again, *"please don't kill anyone, please don't kill anyone."*

There are others, however, who are purposefully and maliciously motivated to be as negative as possible. These individuals have an internal need to be negative, recruit others to their selfish cause, and even work together to sabotage everything that is put in place to create a positive change within their workplace environment. Their intrinsic motivation stems from a previous incident or occurrence that has changed the attitude of this individual. Whether it be a recent disciplinary action, a proposed change that threatens a personal freedom, or something from home that creates a negative feeling within oneself, these negative feelings drive the negative behavior. These individuals are energized by the power of going against the norm, and they create turmoil in order to feel relevant on a team that has either failed to acknowledge them or has chosen not to identify with such behaviors. I call these folks the 20 percenters and we will discuss what to do with them later in the book. Undermining access to self-determination and self-empowerment can also lead to negative intrinsic motivation and working against leadership rather than with it. When freedoms are removed, the caregiver personnel may feel a sense of disempowerment. The strength of the reaction is proportional to the number of choices or privileges removed and their relative importance. This concept is also known as reactance theory (Brehem, 1968).

For instance, if you tell the caregivers that from now on they have to wear black shoes, not white, they'll probably think: *Big deal. I've got to go buy black shoes instead of white.* They might grumble a little, but it's really not a big deal. What if you tell them instead, "As of today you only get 15 minutes for lunch"? There would be a greater negative reaction based on their perception of the importance of the freedom affected. The more important the restriction or change, the greater the reaction.

Restricting a greater number of freedoms will also increase the reaction. For example, if a leadership group got together and said, "We need to make some changes. There's too much texting during work hours, people are on their phones too often and/or there are too many breaks during the day, including smoking breaks. Effective immediately there will be no more texting, personal phone calls, or smoking breaks," there would be a mutiny amongst many of the staff. The reaction may vary based on the importance of those freedoms. The Millennials would be up in arms; however, the Baby Boomers may not protest at all, understanding that two of the freedoms being restricted, texting and phone calls, are not something that is as important to them.

We often see this in action in the workplace. Suppose you have a group of employees who have been able to work collectively to develop their schedules and time off. They've enjoyed this ability—or freedom—and value it highly. Now, in comes a new manager who wants to do things differently. No more group scheduling. The manager is in charge now. What do you think the likely reaction will be? Right. Reactance. And pretty strong reactance, if experience is any guide.

Finally, if there's more than one change try to find a way to space out the changes so that caregivers do not feel like everything is changing at once. For those who fear change, the reaction will increase proportionally to the number of changes happening.

Positive Extrinsic Motivation

Extrinsic motivation represents the forces outside of our own innate desires that affect our behavior. It includes rewards and/or acknowledgments, such as financial rewards (salary and bonuses), promotions, and other signs of appreciation (food provided by leadership during a busy shift).

When the shift is long and busy, good leaders will find a way to motivate staff through that day or shift. Focusing on extrinsic factors is an immediate fulfillment of needs, thus it is an easier motivation tool. The most familiar example of extrinsic motivation is money. When organizations ensure that staff evaluations are truly merit based then higher percentage raises (money) are given to individuals based on their performance. The hope is the reward of money may somehow motivate a person to perform above and beyond their abilities. Although this concept makes sense in relation to extrinsic motivation, what I found is that those who perform the best on evaluations are not inspired by the potential for a bigger raise, but rather driven more by intrinsic factors such as pride or competence. There are some underperformers who are solely motivated by the promise of money, which comes from a very extrinsic and selfish place.

There are times as leaders where extrinsic motivation is necessary and positive. We do these things because they are quick, they are effective in the short term, and they are, quite frankly, the right thing to do. As rewarding as these gestures can be, you will inevitably encounter individuals who do not appreciate the effort. Too much positive reinforcement shown in the same fashion without variety can seem repetitive and, at times, lead caregivers to look beyond the gesture and criticize that nothing is being done to support them. Caregiver perception shifts from positive extrinsic motivation to expected employer responsibility. For example, in the winter, when the population in most hospitals is high, the boarding of inpatients in the emergency department becomes a reality. This can be very stressful and provides an elevated atmosphere for burn out. Since it is a challenge to get everyone to lunch, it is sometimes supplied by leadership as a thank you for their hard work and acknowledgement that they may not get a full lunch. At some point, caregivers will inevitably say, "Pizza again?" switching their perception of the pizza from a gift to an expectation. The easy response is to take it personally. But, leaders should always focus on the reason behind the gesture and not the few who question the intent. Understand that leaders should appreciate the 80 percent that are thankful for the gesture and ignore the 20 percent who don't. Do the right thing because it is simply the right thing to do.

Negative Extrinsic Motivation

Negative extrinsic motivation is when you get the result you are looking for through a negative stimulus. For example, the threat of being written up will help motivate individuals to complete a task in a timely fashion. This is the least desirable form of motivation. Not only does it send message accompanied by a threat, but for a leader, it is exhausting. Remember to write up Jamie. Address Greg's remarks before you leave for the day. Call Grace back because she had an issue with Jacob. Being positive just feels good. It is a choice in healthcare leadership to focus most of the attention on those being negative. We focus on the negative people because they try to dominate our attention.

So why do leaders spend 80 percent of their time on the negative energy people? If you spend 80 percent of our time on the negative people, what percentage of our time do the positive people get? Leaders need to reverse that philosophy and focus on the good people. Spend the majority of your day thanking people and encouraging teamwork. Being positive can be just as contagious as negative energy it just takes a little more effort. Often that positive energy will help to empower the team players and, in turn, help them police the bad people and eventually demand that they change their ways.

Misconceptions

We have spent some time talking about what motivates individuals and how to use that knowledge to help caregivers feel fulfilled and be successful. As important as it is to understand this concept, it is also important to discuss some of the common misconceptions that leaders have as to what does or does not motivate people.

When asked what motivates caregivers, many leaders, and others in healthcare, will be the first to say that it is money that makes their caregivers happy. Raises and bonuses are believed to be the magic solution to ensure caregiver engagement. Have you ever had a job where you dreaded going to work each day, but stayed in that job because the money was too good to pass up? Perhaps you have, but inevitably some day you make a decision the money is not enough.

Money in itself is *not* a motivation—*unless* other intrinsic motivating factors are present. This was demonstrated in a 2004 study by Firth Et.al. and published in the *Journal of Managerial Psychology* describing how managers could reduce employees' intentions to quit.[14] Firth and colleagues asked respondents to answer the following question, "Over the course of your career, what has been the most significant reason you have chosen to leave your employer?" Yes, compensation was a factor in the study but—and it's an important but—it was cited by only 8 percent of the respondents as a precipitating factor. "Lack of excitement" was the primary determining factor when deciding to leave a job, and it was cited by 39 percent of those

---

[14] Firth, l., Mellor, D., Moore, K., & Loquet, C. (2004). How can managers reduce employee intention to quit. Journal of Managerial Psychology, 19, 170-187

surveyed.

Others have studied the importance of pay in relation to overall job satisfaction and found that money was not the predominant reason that employees were dissatisfied or the main reason they left their employer. In 2010 Tim Judge et al. reviewed multiple studies, which encompassed 120 years of research from 92 research studies. Analysis showed a very weak correlation between job satisfaction and money. This comprehensive review showed that many things influence job satisfaction, with money being low on that list.[15] The survey Group Gallup, conducted employee engagement surveys of over 1.4 million employees, from 34 nations, and found that there was "no significant difference in employee engagement by pay level."[16]

Lack of a challenge is a form of showing competence and achievement, both intrinsic motivators. Those who "disagree with corporate culture" have fundamental issues with the philosophy of the company. In other words, their expectations, values, and beliefs are often in conflict. And, an internal sense of achievement is either stunted or in some instances eliminated. Without this internal satisfaction, there is no incentive to work in an effort to benefit the company, or for that matter to benefit ourselves.

USING MOTIVATION TO OUR BENEFIT

It is important to understand caregivers individually in order to fully harness their potential. If a caregiver enjoys working with a team toward a shared goal, then we must find a way to foster and encourage that desire. Perhaps this is a caregiver who you ask to chair the best practice committee. Although leading a group may not be a strength, the idea of joining a team who can make real change may motivate them to accept the challenge of chairperson.

There are some people who thrive when they have the opportunity to show their clinical competence. Acknowledgement of this strength by leadership and their fellow colleagues helps motivate an individual to perform additional tasks. These caregivers are often the ones chosen to

[15] Judge, T.A., Piccolo, R.F., Podsakoff, N.P., Shaw, J.C., Rich, B.L. (2010). The relationship between pay and job satisfaction: A meta analysis of the literature. *Journal of Vocational Behavior*, 77(2). 157-167.

[16] State of the American Workplace. (2013). Retrieved February 2, 2015 from http://employeeengagement.com/wp-content/uploads/2013/06/Gallup-2013-State-of-the-American-Workplace-Report.pdf

precept new bedside caregivers to the department. Why? They are clinically competent, but, more importantly, this task gives them a sense of purpose and allows them to show off a skill that sets them apart from others.

When I first started as an emergency department nurse, I was motivated by this type of challenge. I always tell others that I love emergency medicine because medically you need to know a little bit about everything. But, after a while, that motivation is not enough. I needed a new challenge. So, when a leadership position in the ED became available, I immediately applied. I went through the interview process and subsequently was not given the job. Discouraged, I went to my manager and asked why I was not offered the position. Her simple and quick reply was, "You're not ready."

What did she mean I was not ready? I was an excellent nurse. When someone needed to get that difficult IV stick, they came to me. When they needed a preceptor, they came to me. What did she mean, I'm not ready? She explained to me that being a leader was more than being clinically competent; it was about leading from an emotional, psychological, and clinical perspective. I still didn't understand. I asked what I could do to prove I was ready. She looked up and said, "I will give you something to do." She got out of her chair and took me to one of the treatment rooms. She told me that she wanted all of the drawers in each room to be labeled and to look the same. When finished, I was to report back to her.

Seriously? Label drawers? I begrudgingly did the assigned medial task. After completing I went back to her. "Did you finish what I asked you to do?" I answered yes. She then asked me, "Why did you do what I asked you to do?" I immediately answered her, "Because you told me to." She looked at me and said, "Okay, you're still not ready." My first thought was, *This woman is crazy.*

I continued to be angry for a few weeks. Determined not to give up, I made a decision to show her she was wrong. I found other things to do. Offered suggestions to improve processes. Volunteered for committees. I even dressed up as Santa Claus for the Christmas party. With each completed task came the desire to do more, to be better not for her but for me. I was motivated to show that I was competent as a leader. I deserved the job not because of the clinical skills I possessed but because of the desire I had to make my working environment the best possible. My boss' purpose for assigning me the task to label the drawers was to show me that clinical competence was good but not enough. After completing the task I expected the job. Real learning is not in the task, it is in the "why" I did the task. Once I understood this I was better prepared to lead.

It's important for leaders to understand human behavior and to understand their caregivers as individuals: what are their intrinsic and extrinsic motivations, what are their values, what's important to them and to what degree are those things important.

Creating the Ultimate Working Experience

If you were asked today what the ultimate working experience looks like, what would your answer be? Would it be that you work with a group of people who are always pitching in? Perhaps it is that the fun people are all on at the same time? Some may say that it is when everything during your shift goes smoothly and before you know it the shift is over.

If we asked leaders the same question I believe they would have the same answers, a great team that works together to provide a compassionate and caring patient experience for both patients and their families.

Setting a Values-based Vision Statement

When you use motivation and empowerment as a way to engage the caregivers, real culture change begins to become a possibility. The culture change is not marked by a single event, which makes it difficult to identify, but rather a series of small events that create the ultimate experience. The culture changes and people begin to believe in the system, practice the values, and hold each other accountable for the success of the unit. I am still amazed when bedside caregivers find solutions to issues before I even know there is a problem or when they create a patient experience initiative that I would have never thought of initiating myself. It's what makes me happy as a leader. It's that "aha!" moment when you say, "Yes! We changed the culture!"

How then do you get everyone to be on the same page? If you want caregivers to follow you they need to know where they are going. What is expected of them and what can they expect from you? What is the groups expectations and vision for the future of the department?

For years organizations have relied on mission statements to unite their workforce and give them a sense of purpose. In nursing school, I remember being given an assignment to develop a mission statement during a nursing leadership course. Even then, I remembered struggling to try to come up with a few lines that would be general enough to include everyone and yet specific enough to help provide a vision that is relevant and important to all. It's nearly impossible.

Despite its downfalls, almost every healthcare institution uses mission statements. My thought? They don't work. Don't believe me? Go to work tomorrow, ask the first 10 people you see what their mission statement is, and then ask them to recite it for you. If I was a betting man, I would guess most of them will get it wrong. Even when you teach nursing, the simple mention of mission statements puts the audience immediately to sleep. You can just see it in their eyes.

Why does this happen? Who often makes these statements? Senior leadership? Marketing? Do they ask the caregivers who work at the bedside for their opinion? Most leaders don't. Do they ask them what they believe is the right thing for patients? Wouldn't it make sense to ask? I mean these caregivers spend 24 hours a day caring for the patients, yet they are often excluded from the creation of the mission statement, which is supposed to define the care they are asked to deliver.

Now, I know there are purists out there who believe in mission statements. I, too, believe they hold some value from an organizational perspective; however, I believe that if you want the caregivers' buy-in, you have to ask the caregivers what is important to them. When bedside caregivers feel valued and when they have a say in the vision and rules of the department, they are more likely to commit to that set of values.

It is easy to find examples of this type of philosophy when it comes to creating an employee driven business model. I often quote Herb Kelleher, the founder of Southwest Airlines, because he understood the value of getting the employees opinions and ideas and ultimately their loyalty. He made sure that his employees were engaged and understood that this was imperative if the company had a chance to compete with other airlines. His philosophy was that all employees should have a say.

Engaged caregivers want the culture to be positive and supportive. They want the team to be successful. You just need to give them the opportunity. Allow them the freedom to speak up and thank them when they do. If they make a mistake, ensure them that it is okay and then look for the opportunity to learn from it and then find the opportunity for improvement. Empower the people, and they will do wonderful things.

Game Plan Tip: Clinical Excellence Commitment Boards

A Clinical Excellence Commitment board encapsulates a group of philosophies or rules bedside caregivers develop to create a place where patients receive the best care possible and where the caregivers create the ultimate working experience. Everyone on your unit, everyone who is part of the team, techs, unit clerks, nursing assistants, PAs, physicians—everyone has a say. It unites a group and helps them to define what the vision of the department looks like and the culture it hopes to create.

Step 1: The first step is to simply give everyone a 5 x 8 index card and answer the two questions below. The purpose is to isolate behaviors or personality traits that each caregiver believes is important to ensuring the best team possible. This can be a positive statement like "I enjoy working with people who work together as a team." Or the caregiver can list what they don't want. "I don't like working with people who are always late for work." Why do we list the negatives? Simple, it is as important to know the things we want to avoid in future caregiver personnel, as well as the characteristics that we do want. There are no right or wrong responses, only the feeling or thoughts of the individuals that are delivering them.

> ➤ On one side of the card, answer this question:
>   - Describe the ultimate working experience, one where you walk into the department, look at your team, and say to yourself, "This is going to be a great day!"
> ➤ On the other side of the card, answer the question:
>   - Describe the ultimate healing experience where you can leave your mother or child overnight in the department and know they are in great hands.

Step 2: Gather up all of the cards. Go through them, read what they've said, and start to identify trends. You might get 15 different people saying something similar in 15 different ways. Put similar thoughts together in piles and then assign a value to the pile. Maybe you create a pile for teamwork, a pile for respect, or a pile for commitment—whatever the themes might be.

Step 3: For each pile of cards, find one specific verbatim comment that sums up the sentiment of all of the similar thoughts. Using the comment, verbatim, helps the bedside caregivers see their work in the process. I guarantee that when you pull your caregivers back together to look at the board they're going to be looking for their statements, their sentiments. When they see their words they will be sure to let the other caregivers know that they are their words thus ensuring that this process is truly about them.

Step 4: Take each statement and start to create a clinical excellence commitment board by numbering them. These should be limited to no more than 20 and at least 10. This statement board should be placed on a poster and laminated. (Recommended: 4 foot by 3 foot poster board.)

Step 5: At the bottom of each standards board, add a statement that reads, "I agree that the above statements are not rules, but a philosophy, a commitment to my fellow caregivers. This is a philosophy I am willing to accept. I want to make the ICU (or whatever your unit is) the best unit, a place where caregivers enjoy coming to work and where patients love the care they receive. I will practice this philosophy every hour, every shift, every day."

Step 6: Have a commitment party and celebrate. Bring everyone together. Have them read it, and then give them a sharpie and ask them to sign it as a sign of their commitment. Everyone is required to sign if you are to be a part of the unit. Do this for everyone. No one should be excluded. If they refuse, ask them why and then insist that they sign. This is the entire team's vision for the department. Not leadership's vision it is the caregivers vision. If they decided not to contribute ideas for the board that was their decision, but the expectation is they will follow what the unit wants. If you don't want to sign, you need to explain why to your colleagues.

Step 7: After everyone has signed it, find a place where patients, families, and colleagues can see it. Be proud. Post it for all to see.

Step 8: Create a paper version of the standards and provide it to all new employees before they interview. "Welcome to your interview. Before we get started I want you to read something. These are our Clinical Excellence Commitment Standards. This is our philosophy, and is the vision for our department. This is who we are. It is our culture. I want to make sure you feel comfortable with these commitment standards and, if you do, we can proceed with the interview. If not, I understand and we respect that, but this is probably not the place for you to work."

Case Study

When we did this for my ER, we had 14 Clinical Excellence Commitment Standards. As we unveiled the board at our commitment ceremony, people gravitated to the board, some staring at it longer than others in order find their statement within the comments. I remember one particular nursing assistant standing in front of the board, calling others over to the board saying "Look at number eleven!! That's from my card." Her idea for the board? "Treat everyone with respect regardless of their job title." That is what was important to her. And, based on the number of people listening to her boast, it was important to them as well. There was an excitement in the room. Culture building process started!

Other comments that were chosen included:

- "When needed, ask for assistance and accept it when offered." The reason for this standard? "There are some nurses that are really nasty, and when you offer to help them, they say, 'no, I don't need your help'. I just stopped being nice to her."
- "Be on time and ready for report. After 12 long hours, you would want the same thing. To go home!" Apparently, this was an issue. Some caregivers would routinely come in late while others would come in right at change of shift, but then would spend 10 minutes at their locker getting ready. Because this was identified as a clinical standard, it then became apparent that it wasn't fair and that it needed to change.

This caregiver-driven initiative has to be respected because it is about the team and not the individual. The rules didn't come from management; it came from their peers.

As a leader, there are ways, to interject some of your own desires for colleague behavior into the standards. You are a part of the team as well and should not be excluded. When the cards are collected only you, the manager, or leadership team, should collect the data. Most of the standards will come from bedside caregivers, but I added one or two standards that I felt would make a better unit. For example, I wanted caregivers to play a greater part in the decisions that affected the unit. So, we started a self-governance system. Attendance was good, but not as good as it could be. So, I took the opportunity to add my standard to the board. "I will offer my ideas in a creative way by attending my committee meetings and by being a part of the solution."

These boards started just in the ER. But the power of the people spread. You can now find commitment boards in the ICU, Telemetry units, and the progressive care unit. Even the radiology department has one, and they say it has been instrumental in unifying caregivers and improving their scores. Each one is unique to the needs of the unit and the desires of the caregivers.

Using The Clinical Excellence Commitment Board to Set the Tone

When new hires come on board they go through an onboarding process. All new employees, regardless of discipline or unit, come to the onboarding class. During that process, I talk about our standards and what's expected of them. In a traditional orientation, the caregivers spend a lot of time talking about clinical standards, as well as policies and procedures, but never talk about the behavioral expectations or philosophy of the unit. This is critical to the success of the individual and as a leader you cannot expect behavior if the caregiver is not aware of the expectations.

The first day on the job after onboarding, we introduce the new caregiver, welcome them, give them a Sharpie, and take them over to the clinical excellence commitment board, which they're asked to sign. After that occurs we again welcome them, thank them, and they are officially now part of the team.

Leadership should help create the Clinical Excellence Commitment Board collaboratively and use it as a motivation tool as well as a way to have all caregivers understand the unit expectations.

If an issue needs to be addressed, pull the colleague to the board, find the standard that applies to the infraction, and ask them to read it. Follow up with the question "Did you meet that commitment standard?" After a while you will start to see caregivers pulling other caregivers over to the board and holding them accountable for their actions. The 80 percent will rise up and hold the 20 percent accountable. Who can argue with commitment standards that your fellow colleagues created and you signed? The answer: *No one.* It's powerful. It's symbolic. And it works.

Finding the Intrinsically Motivated

Understanding now that intrinsically motivated individuals are better caregivers, we must find a way to identify them during the interview process. Discovering and interviewing potential bedside caregivers who are intrinsically motivated can be difficult. People practice interview skills. There are hundreds of sources that can help to coach prospective interviewees in the art of interviewing.

There is no exact science to finding the right team. There are many books that speak to identifying behaviors or studying resumes to find that highly motivated individual, however I have found success by going back to what I believe is key to creating the ultimate working environment and that is staying true to the caregiver commitment standards that the caregivers create themselves. There is an underlying value assigned to each of the standards. When interviewing perspective caregivers, we use value-centered questions to determine if the person is a fit. For example, one of the standards that seems to be present in many of the Clinical Excellence Commitment boards I have helped create is "I will treat everyone with respect, regardless of their job title." This standard helps each caregiver understand that we do not talk about job titles, we only refer to each other as team members. Each job that is performed provides value to the patient experience, thus all jobs are important. So the value assigned to this standard is "respect".

Understanding that this value of respect is what the caregivers want in the people who work next to them, we then must make up an interview question that specifically assesses the value in the interviewee. For example a question may be "Tell me about an experience in work or in your life where you felt someone was disrespected and then tell me what you felt and how you handled it." Allow the individual the opportunity to think about the question. Allow for silence after the question is asked and fight the urge to help the person answer the question. It is the poise of the person as they think about the answers as much as it is the answer itself. Do this for each value identified. Keep the questions open-ended, and avoid yes no answers.

I always like to throw in a question they don't expect and watch their reaction. For example I'll ask them, "Tell me something you do simply because it's fun." Or, "What is the name of your favorite recipe, and why do you like it?" In these questions, the answers are irrelevant. What I look for is the sureness of the answer. Someone that is confidant in who they are will be confident in the role they assume on your team.

True caregiver engagement takes some time to achieve and based on experience it is very easy to get lost along the way. Caregivers will test your patience, and if not kept in check, your frustration and emotions will destroy your own motivation for wanting to change the culture. Motivation plays such a central role in the process of culture change. Remember the formula of Motivation x Empowerment = Caregiver Engagement to guide your journey and keep you on track.

CHAPTER 3
DARING TO TRUST

DEVELOPING CREDIBILITY AS A LEADER

Leadership credibility and trust are built over time. Caregivers will watch everything that you do and, at times, even test some of the things that you say. They know when you leave work early or come in late. They will figure out that you didn't enforce a policy for someone you like, but did enforce it with someone you do not like. Being truthful, respecting caregiver's rights, and being consistent in your behavior will help to build your credibility as a leader. These are vital steps needed to build healthy relationships with caregivers. As a new leader, this takes time. For the experienced leader, it takes patience and the ability to say to yourself maybe the way things are today isn't working.

First Things First: Know Thyself

Before asking others to abide by the rules and be true to the vision of the department, a leader must follow the rules and model the behaviors themselves. You cannot control your own behavior, however, if you are not aware that it exists. Knowing yourself involves a personal journey where you explore your needs, your emotions, your pet peeves, your weaknesses, and your strengths. Understanding your own tendencies can help you regulate emotions and responses to difficult situations. Like change, knowing yourself is not a one-time event. It is a lifetime of self-awareness.[17]

---

[17] Goleman, D. (1995). *Emotional intelligence: Why it can matter more than IQ.* New

Game Plan Tip: Get to Know Me Grid

How do you as a leader get to know your own behaviors? Here's a simple exercise you can do; it's something I like to do in my workshops.

1. Take a sheet of paper and divide it into 4.
2. Write the words "Strengths," "Weaknesses," "Needs," and "Pet Peeves" in the boxes. For example:

Strengths	Weaknesses
Needs	Pet Peeves

3. In each box fill in how your own behavior is demonstrated. Think hard, be honest with yourself, and create your lists. What are you good at? What do you think other people think you're good at? What makes you an effective leader? Take these characteristic traits and list them under the strengths column.
4. Next, do the same thing for the weakness column. What areas could you improve in? What might others think your weaknesses are? When I do this in my workshops, I am always amazed that the section leaders have the greatest trouble filling out is the strengths section. We are so much better at being critical of ourselves then we are at paying ourselves compliments. Be brave. If you want the exercise to be beneficial, then you must be honest with yourself.

York: Bantam.

5. Continue by filling out the needs section. What do you, as an individual, need in order to succeed? What motivates you? What does it take to make you feel happy and satisfied?

6. Finally, list your pet peeves. What really bugs you? What behaviors or actions really test your resolve as a leader when someone presents them in front of you? These are really important to identify, not because you can stop the behavior, but because when the behavior or action is present you will need to regulate your emotions and reactions to remain in control.

7. Now comes the difficult part. After you have completed the grid, open yourself to others' opinions. Quite often our opinions of ourselves do not match what others see. Take that piece of paper and give it to someone you respect or that you feel knows you the best. First, ask them if they agree with your list. Be sure to tell them that you need them to be honest. Then ask them what they would add to the list. Choose the right person to help you. Be open to their suggestions. Be open to honest feedback.

8. Next, give them a copy of your list and ask them to point it out to you when you're exhibiting your strengths and, more importantly, when you're displaying your weaknesses. It takes real courage to ask for constructive criticism, and even more to have someone point out your flaws. Real growth comes from this kind of feedback and openness with yourself that there is always room for improvement.

Case Study

When I was the manager of an Emergency Department, I asked my leadership team to join me in this exercise. I gave them my piece of paper and I said, "Guys, I need you to tell me, your boss, when I'm doing these things on my list, especially my weaknesses, because I need to get better at them." They agreed to provide me with feedback. In turn, they shared their lists with me.

One of the weaknesses that they identified was my tendency to combine a compliment with the word "but." I would say something like "You did a really good job, but" rather than simply ending with the positive acknowledgment. If I wanted to improve as a leader, I needed to eliminate the "buts." I told them, "We need to have a code word that we can use when I use a "but" in public because I don't want you to just shout out "Chuck, you just said 'but' again!". So, I suggested that we use a code word that only we knew. I choose the word "Colorado."

A few days later we put the process to the test. It was nurses' week and we decided to have a contest for the caregivers. We asked them to help create a visual representation, a logo, which we could use on correspondence, paperwork, etc. that represented the ER. We asked caregivers to come up with ideas for a logo that would encompass the five values of our department. The best logo entered would win a prize. We started getting some entries, but nothing that was exceptional; nothing stood out. Then, one day, one of my clinical leads came to me and said, "Look at this!" She handed me a drawing that I felt encompassed everything we were looking for. I wanted to know who had created it, so she said, "Follow me; you're never going to believe this."

We walked out to the unit, and she took me up to one of our environmental services staff and said, "Charles, let me introduce you to Sam. Sam wasn't sure she could submit something for the contest because she's not one of the ER staff."

I remember Sam was apologetic, and she seemed unsure if she was going to get in trouble for submitting a logo. I asked her to tell me about her design and what she was thinking. She told me her vision and I replied while referring directly to the logo itself, "You know, I really like how you've displayed the pillars and the values. I love the way the hallway leads to the doors of the ER. But, the only thing I'm concerned about is that you included the hospital values as well, which I think is a little confusing."

"Colorado! Colorado!"

What had I done? I had just taken a good opportunity to provide positive feedback to a caregiver and I blew it. I immediately knew that I'd messed up. My clinical lead soon pulled me to the side and said, "Charles, you were talking to her and she was so excited that you accepted her entry, and then you butted her and I watched her face go from excitement and appreciation to deflation."

Oh no, I had done it again! The difference though was that this time I had an opportunity to correct the mistake soon after it had happened. Before I had allowed myself to be open to criticism, that conversation would have happened and nothing positive would have come from it. Instead, an introspective review of my own weakness allowed me to grow as a leader. That's progress, that's power.

I knew I needed to apologize, and I did. I walked out to the department, found Sam, and said, "Sam, I apologize. You didn't have to do this. You did a wonderful job, better than anybody else who's submitted an idea, and I'm going to submit it as is." I did and her design was selected.

Realize your weakness and capitalize on your strengths. Have the courage and be open enough to receive feedback from others even when the focus is on your flaws. That one opportunity helped me to grow as a person and as a leader.

Earn Their Trust

In order to earn the trust of others, leaders must be consistent in their behaviors and honest in their approach. Self-accountability to the standards set for the department is again the first step. It starts with you. It starts at the top. Your caregivers need to know that you're not somebody who rules from behind a desk. They need to know that you're working with them and willing to do the same things that you're asking them to do, and not doing the things you've asked them not to do. If you tell someone that "texting is not allowed on the unit," and then 10 minutes later, they see you texting, you will immediately lose credibility and, ultimately, their trust.

One way to build trust with caregivers is to first trust them. Yes, I understand that trusting blindly can be dangerous. And yes, in the beginning some caregivers could possibly take advantage of that trust. But once mutual trust is established then respecting that ideal becomes a central focus of everyone who is part of the culture that you have established. It becomes the glue or the foundation so to speak for the department. When I first assumed the role of leader, I tried to use trust as a way of showing my support to the caregivers. I remember the following conversation. "Charles, I'm just devastated. My godchild's christening is on the 16th and I didn't know I was working and have tried everybody to try to get off, but I haven't been able to find anyone," I did what I could do to help that person arrange coverage. That kind of support is appreciated, not just by that caregiver, but by others who are observing and know that you will do the same for them. It builds a solid relationship between a leader and the caregivers.

The job caregivers do every day is very difficult, and they need the support of their leader. So, do it and be supportive. When a caregiver comes to you with an issue, don't second guess. Don't judge. Listen. Then, offer support: "How can I help you with this?" or "How can I provide you with the resources you need?" Be genuine. I don't know how to say this but you have to want to help them. That starts with an internal drive or desire to be a helpful person, which has to come naturally. It must be organic. If you find that you need to force yourself to find the compassion to empathize with their issues, then perhaps you need to ask if leadership is the right job for you.

If you have decided that leadership is what you want to do, then be sincere. Even when the caregivers bring issues to you that you believe are inconsequential, it's important that you provide an objective sounding board. Remember everyone's issues are relative and real to them. They are living with the issue, and despite our personal feelings, we need to understand that for them the issue is very important, regardless of how minimal you may believe it to be.

Creating a positive culture relies on a foundation of trust. Trust among fellow caregivers as well as the trust that is developed between caregivers and their leader. There are additional requirements for building trust, which include:

> Setting clear expectations
> Being consistent
> Being timely
> Avoiding playing favorites
> Being discreet

Set Clear Expectations

A leader must define what is expected of each and every caregiver. If caregivers do not know what is expected of them, then frustration will occur when rules are broken or policies violated. The responsibility, however, falls on the leader. They must find a way to not only define the expectation, but also find a way to get everyone to follow what has been set as the expectation. Caregivers can't succeed if they don't know what is expected of them.

When you are defining expectations, you need to make the caregivers a part of that process similarly to when we are trying to include caregivers in the culture change process. Not only will you have buy-in, but eventually you will see self-accountability because they want to see what they created be successful. It stems from pride and an internal motivation. Using the

Clinical Excellence Commitment board allows you and the caregivers to define expectations and then hold each other accountable.

Be Consistent

Being consistent as a leader helps provide a stable work environment where people understand that they are all being held accountable to the same standards. You cannot discipline one person for something and then ignore that same action from another. Keep in mind that each caregiver is always watching you to ensure that you are being fair. They're always watching! They will test you to see how you react to certain situations and how you treat certain individuals. This is particularly the case when it comes to new leaders. The positive caregivers will test you to see if you're different from other leaders they have experienced who didn't listen to them. The negative ones will test you to see what they can get away with or to see how they can manipulate you to get what they want. They will notice right away if you're giving some preference to another caregiver or not following the standards consistently.

For example, let's say that you create a new policy and cover it during one of your caregiver huddles. During your Monday morning huddle, you say, "Hey, guys, I have to tell you that texting has gotten a little out of hand. What we need you to do is if you need to text someone do it in the break room or in the restroom. You cannot be texting in public." Message delivered.

Then on Tuesday, you're on the unit and you see somebody texting, but you're really, really busy and don't have the time to stop and correct the behavior. So, you walk on by without saying a word.

What have you just done? You've, in effect, given the other 20 people who saw you walk past the person permission to text in public. The next day you see that same behavior and have the time to address it, but you unfortunately can't because you run the risk of caregivers seeing you as being inconsistent and playing favorites. You have now lost the right to correct the behavior. The big takeaway: when you see something being done that violates some policy, value, or norm you must act. Inaction on your part is interpreted as permission on the part of the other caregivers. One of my favorite quotes that I live by when it comes to being consistent is from a good friend, Dr. Jay Kaplan. He puts it very simply, "If you permit it, you promote it." Remember, *they are always watching*. You must be consistent.

Be Timely

It's important that leaders address issues in a timely fashion. Regardless of how busy you are, we've already seen the damage that can be done when you choose to ignore—even for a while—some behavior that is clearly violating some rule, some policy, or some expectation.

Will there be situations where you literally do not have the time to deal with the issue at that moment? Yes. But, if we think about the texting situation, regardless of how busy you are, you can say something like: "Hey, no texting; put that away," and then go back later to a more in-depth conversation.

It's important, though, that you do this follow up as quickly as you possibly can. If the texting incident happened on a Monday, and you don't address it until Friday, that's not a timely response, and the conversation loses its sense of importance.

Don't Play Favorites

Playing favorites is one of the quickest ways to lose the trust and credibility of the caregivers. We need to make a distinction here, however, between *having* favorites and *playing* favorites. It seems logical that you would favor your best employees and disfavor the poor performers. When you play favorites, the implication is that an individual is receiving preferential treatment based on nothing more than personal opinion. This subjective point-of-view can be detrimental to building trust among all the caregivers. However, those who *become favorites* do so by consistently exceeding expectations and positively contributing to the culture of the department. It is based on objective information and an individual's professional productivity.

People who step up to take on extra responsibility, who go above and beyond expectations, are going to be my favorites. It is a reward for going the extra mile. For always trying to exceed the expectation. You should be rewarded, and I should do everything possible to help make your work environment the best possible. You earn the right to be a favorite.

I often say to those who question my integrity that the power to be a favorite is in one person's control...theirs. "If you want to be a favorite, prove that you are here for your colleagues and your department, not just here for yourself." Be a favorite by stepping up and positively contributing. Come up with ideas. Look for solutions to problems. Be a positive influence. Show me that you are willing to do more than what's expected in order to positively contribute to our department. When you do that, then you, too, will be one of my favorites.

One word of caution, be sure to hold everyone, including "favorites," accountable to the rules and expectations and be consistent with the consequences that have been enforced in the past. When you blur that line and ignore behaviors, then yes you are now playing favorites. All caregivers need to be held to the same expectations.

Keep Your Composure

Like any other leader, you will find that there are those topics that just set you off. They are your list of pet peeves that when presented in front of you will require extra vigilant composure and restraint. You, however, must maintain your composure at all times. I know it is difficult sometimes but I have never met an angry leader that was respected by their caregivers.

Leaders are however human beings. Maintaining your composure, at times, is a mental exercise, and it's something that you, personally, will need to master. There are many leadership skills that you can learn from a book, a conference, or from a mentor, but there are some skills that you personally have to work on; this is one of them.

This coping process is a two-step process. The first step is keeping your composure. The second step, which proves to be an even greater feat, is masking your true feelings or emotions so that others aren't able to read what's going on in your mind. That requires being cognizant of the nonverbal cues you may be sending. In the next chapter, we discuss using your communication skills to be an effective leader, but it truly can be an exhausting skill to perfect.

Keeping your composure is paramount when getting your point across effectively. You need to maintain control—of the situation and of yourself. The minute you "lose it," you're out of the game.

Be Discreet

Sometimes despite your best efforts, there will be a caregiver who doesn't believe in the direction the department is heading and a conversation is needed. You have spoken to the caregiver about their behavior and now everyone is on the same page about expectations. You are with a group of other leaders in the cafeteria, and you are talking to them about the conversation you just had. Someone overhears you and reports back to the caregiver about the boss's indiscretion regarding what was intended as a private conversation. Credibility gone. Trust is gone. You are back to square one.

As a leader you will have sensitive, and, at times emotional, conversations with caregivers and, sometimes, you may be tempted to share those experiences with others. Let me be clear, although leaders are supposed to set a higher standard, they themselves are human beings with emotions of their own and at times, they need to vent their frustrations. These venting sessions cannot be conducted in a public setting. It's disrespectful to the caregiver. If you need reminding, just think about a time when that happened to you. Your trust is betrayed. It stinks, and you wouldn't want it to happen to you, so don't do it to them. If you feel you need collegial support, do it the right way, in private, behind closed doors, and with a trusted colleague.

Follow the Chain of Command

Building trust occurs at all levels, caregiver to caregiver, leader to caregiver, and leader to leader. Following the chain of command is imperative when it comes to managing problems or concerns. As a leader, you want to trust that the caregivers are telling you when they are frustrated or angry. This is easier to do when you have established that trust is mutual between leader and caregiver. Unfortunately, there are some leaders who don't understand the importance of this concept.

I had a boss that did this to me all the time. When you start a new job and change is needed, caregiver frustration can occur. Open communication is important to establish between the leader and colleague. My boss, however, didn't see the importance. He had an office next to mine and the caregivers would just bypass my office, head straight into his, and shut the door and talk about me. I don't blame them. He set the precedent that he would entertain issues about me as a leader without coming to me first. The caregivers understood this and would take advantage of it. He never turned anyone away, requesting that they speak to the person they had the issue with, *me*. It completely undermined my authority and broke down any kind of trust or credibility that I had developed.

Quite frankly, I was not happy working for an individual who didn't appreciate or value me enough to protect my authority by saying to those individuals, "Hey, I prefer you go directly to Charles first about this." By listening to caregivers, and their complaints, he was allowing staff to overstep my authority.

This same principle applies in caregiver-to-caregiver conversations. I have people all the time that come to me and say, "I'm really mad at Nancy for what she just did." I'll reply, "Did you talk to Nancy?" If the answer is no, I redirect them and inform them they can come back after they have that conversation if they need additional information or support. I only had to do that a few times before they stopped coming to me first and started addressing each other directly. They—and you—need to follow the chain of command.

GET THEIR ATTENTION

Earlier in the chapter, we discussed that caregivers respect a leader who is willing to do anything that caregivers are asked to do. A willingness to step up in times of need to help the department conveys a sense of understanding. If mutual respect exists, the opposite should also be true. Caregivers should understand why a leader is asking for them to do something. Creating that mutual understanding is important. Let me give you an example of how I grabbed the attention of a group of untrusting caregivers early in my leadership career.

In 2001, I joined the caregivers as the manager of the ED. I was from the outside. Hired to repair the reputation of the ED and to improve the care provided to the community, I soon discovered why there were so many problems. This was a very untrusting group who believed the way they were doing things was the right way. In the previous 5 years, they had 4 managers who joined the ED and then quickly departed, not able to handle the group. I was a new leader and people were watching me, testing my limits to see how long before I would quit.

I can tell you that there were lots of challenges, but there were also plenty of opportunities to gain their trust and respect. One such opportunity presented itself on a day when there were a number of call outs. In order to be helpful, I put on my scrubs and assumed the charge nurse role. On this busy day, the waiting room was full and there were patients waiting for up to 4 hours to be seen. As I worked with the caregivers to get patients into open rooms, I noticed that Room 8 was empty, a patient had just left, and the room was dirty. I gave the staff the benefit of the doubt and waited to see if they were going to fill the room. After 10 minutes, I noted that Room 8 was still empty. We had 20 people in the waiting room. I said to one of the nurses, "Hey, we need to bring another patient back to Room 8," and the response was, "Yeah, I know. We called housekeeping. We're just waiting for them to come over and clean it." Say what?

An opportunity! I had a choice. I could get angry and say, "Hey, get off your butt and go do it," or I could seize the opportunity to get their attention. I walked to the other side of the Emergency Department without saying a word, and I found the housekeeping cart. I grabbed a broom and a dustpan, and I walked into Room 8, and started cleaning it.

I still remember the looks on their faces. Like they were all witnessing the discovery of a new species of fish found at the very depths of the ocean. What is he doing? They couldn't believe it. He's in there cleaning up! Why is he cleaning up? That's housekeeping's job. Nope. Not anymore!

Setting the example by displaying the expected behaviors is very powerful. When people see that you are willing to go above and beyond, when you are willing to take on a custodial task to ensure that patients get care delivered as quickly as possible, you take away everyone else's excuse the next time something like that happens. The expectation is set without ever saying a word. Have you ever worked with a leader who was always asking you to do something that they themselves were not willing to do? Defeating isn't it. Empower staff to do the right thing by setting the right example.

Don't Be Afraid to Say You're Sorry

Another way to grab their attention is by admitting that you are human. It always amuses me when I meet leaders who are afraid to admit when they are wrong. "It's a sign of weakness" or "Leaders can't make mistakes". Truth is they do make mistakes and sometimes a lot of them. Admitting your mistake shows that you are willing to admit your failure. Ken Blanchard refers to this as being a vulnerable leader, a point that he drives home in his book *The Servant Leader*. I agree with Blanchard that, as a leader, one of the most powerful things that you can do is show caregivers that you are not perfect—that you too can make, and recover from, errors and missteps.[18]

Caregivers want to know that you are someone who makes mistakes—

---

[18] Autry, J. A., (2001). *The Servant Leader: How to build a creative team, develop great morale, and improve bottom-line performance.* New York, NY: Three Rivers Press.

and is willing to admit it. Not only does it make them feel that you're a human being and can, therefore, understand them when they make mistakes, but it also gives them permission to make mistakes and come forward with them. They know that they will not be penalized for admitting they did something wrong and that the culture of the department is forgivng and understanding.

Leaders need to be vulnerable. They need to be able to say "it's my fault." They need to be able to apologize and accept the responsibility.

Understand the Hot Topic Issues

Credibility can be gained when caregivers believe that you understand their challenges and the issues that affect their daily practice. Understanding what these hot topics are can give you an advantage as a leader by allowing you to address issues that have not been elevated beyond the caregiver level. Identifying an issue and fixing it before anybody even brings it to your attention will communicate to the caregivers that you care about what they care about. It also relays that you are a leader who is present.

Wanting to know the hot topics and finding out what the hot topics are two separate goals. Unfortunately, these caregiver conversations often happen behind closed doors or in small groups huddled together in the corner of the room. The more trust you can establish with the caregivers the higher the chances that these issues are brought to your attention before they escalate into bigger problems.

If hot topic issues are brought to you by a caregiver make sure that the conversation is related to issues and not people. Live the values and expectations of the department even when the conversation is done behind closed doors.

REPAIRING TRUST

The focus of this chapter has been building trust between caregivers and their leaders. The formation of a trusting relationship can take months, if not years, to nurture but only takes one event to destroy it all. When caregivers feel like they can't trust their leader, then they may become cynical and the care will suffer. Words can be hollow if not followed up by the appropriate actions. Unfortunately, there is no quick fix to reestablish that trust. A plan must be established.

➤ First, learn to say you're sorry. Admit the mistake and apologize.

> ➤ Second, accept the responsibility for whatever occurred. You can't hide from it, so get out in front of it.
> ➤ Finally, be humble. Set the example and use the opportunity to improve.

Slowly repair trust by chipping away at what I call the low-hanging fruit, which are the small things you can do immediately to show staff that you want to build trust again. Doing the quick and easy fixes helps immediately show trust while the more difficult challenges can be handled at a later date. This is particularly important if the caregivers had a previous leader that did a lot of promising without a lot of action. Find those 1 or 2 things that you can do immediately and fix them as soon as you can. You have to capture their attention to start the healing process and begin the culture transformation.

An example of this occurred during one of the town hall meetings that I started when I first became the manager of the department. Town hall meetings are an excellent tool to find this low-hanging fruit. I was asked to lead a department where the previous leader had made promises that were never kept. I understood why the caregivers felt cynical. The trust had been broken, and I realized that it would take a serious effort to repair it. I needed to win the caregivers trust back, so I started by meeting with all of the caregivers. Day, night, weekend, weekday, it didn't matter; I met with everyone. I asked them one simple question. What can I do to make your job easier?

I received lots of feedback. Suggestions for improvement, greatest frustrations, and requests for equipment and supplies that they felt they needed. I made a list and then prioritized it showing three categories. What can be fixed now, what needs committee focus to complete, and a third category that I believed I wouldn't be able to change (honesty from a leader can help). The list was posted that same day. I quickly took the low-hanging fruit list and immediately checked off three items from the list. One of the issues identified by the caregivers was that the short nurses could not reach the top shelf in the storage room. A simple fix and a great opportunity to get an easy win.

That day after the meeting, I got into my car, drove to Home Depot, and bought two step ladders. While the caregiver that had presented me with the actual issue was still working, I made an appearance, walked right through the department with my step ladders, and put them in the storage rooms. Without using a word, my message was delivered. I was serious about making positive change.

Think about any relationship that you have ever had in your life. Whether it be a friendship, romantic one, or a working relationship, trust plays an important role in the quality of the connection you have with the other person. Each leader needs to create that trust in order to create a working environment where caregivers are happy to be engaged in the culture change that is occurring. Building trust takes time, but if you are persistent, the payoff will be highly engaged caregivers who work hard for you and the department to create a caring and compassionate healing environment for patients and their families.

CHAPTER 4
CAN I GET A HUGGLE, PLEASE?

COMMUNICATING WITH STAFF

There are three ways that we communicate with others; most of us tend to just think of two—verbal and non-verbal communication. But, there is a third that we will discuss called paraverbal communication. It is important as a leader to understand each level, not only to understand how others communicate, but also to use these skills to communicate to others what you want them to hear. This can be done with purpose, however without monitoring, one can send messages that were otherwise unintended. Being a good communicator is like any other leadership skill, it must be taught, practiced and continually evaluated for its effectiveness. Let's discuss each level of communication, its characteristics, and the potential barriers to achieving successful communication skills.

Verbal Communication

What It Is

Simply put, verbal communication includes both the spoken and written words that we use. It consists of the words we speak and hear, as well as the words that we read and write. For many years linguists have studied language to identify how messages are communicated. But, what influence do the words have on the meaning of the sentence in which they reside? Many argue that the words themselves are only a small portion of the overall message being communicated. Perhaps the most famous to demonstrate this is Dr. Albert Mehrabian, professor emeritus at the University of California-Los Angeles. In 1971, Dr. Mehrabian wrote about his observations of sales people and how they were communicating their sales messages. He believed that messages that were received by customers were 7 percent from the words that they used while the majority of the message, 38 percent from body language and 55 percent from tone of voice, came from the unspoken word.[19] Although others refute this study for overstating the importance of nonverbal communication, many use it as the basis for defining human communication.

Despite the low percentage, words still play a vital role in language. Think of them as the foundation for a house, and nonverbal and paraverbal communication is the actual structure of the house it sits upon. Words help define the thought, which then allows a person to inject nonverbal and paraverbal communication into the statement and bring life to the message. The words you choose could relay the type of leader or caregiver you are, or help form a person's opinion as to who they believe you are. So, choose your words wisely.

Barriers to Verbal Communication

There are many barriers to good communication. When we talk about verbal communication, the most obvious barrier would be education, both the patient's and our own. Mastering the English language can be difficult and choosing the right words to echo a particular sentiment has its challenges. This is particularly difficult when it comes to choosing words when speaking to patients. As a caregiver, how many times have you had to translate what the doctor just said for a patient? Avoid medical jargon, commonly used abbreviations, and complicated medical terms to help prevent confusion.

Another barrier to verbal communication is the pronunciation of words. Caregivers who speak with a strong accent or perhaps in a way that they have been socially or culturally raised, can sometimes be misunderstood. Caregivers must consciously acknowledge this potential barrier and be cognizant of it as they are enunciating their words. This same challenge is apparent when communication is occurring with a person who does not speak the native language. Even when English is the primary language, the difference in the meaning of words can cause confusion. For example, the

[19] Mehrabian, A. (1971). *Silent Messages*. Belmont, CA: Wadsworth.

word "conk" is a term that the British use to refer to their nose. They may use the term lugholes when referencing their ears. Did you know that in Australia they refer to a paper cut as a "guillotine"? Many misconceptions can occur when we are unaware of a word's true or intended meaning.

The final barrier is time. Perhaps the most overlooked barrier, it is the one that most directly affects our ability as caregivers to deliver the right messages. Bedside caregivers often are forced to get their message across in as few words as possible. Unfortunately, time dictates those decisions. Caregivers often have to get to the point with patients and move to the next task. In these fast-paced conversations, caregivers use the fewest words possible to make a point, which can leave a lot of room for patient interpretation.

Keys to Effective Verbal Communication

So, we understand the barriers and agree that choosing the words we use is an important step to effective communication. Now what things do we need to consider to effectively use verbal communication? The most obvious step is to know who you are trying to communicate with. Do they speak your language? Are they cognitively impaired and unable to understand what you are saying? Can they read what you've written? I was told once by a marketing director, while working on a brochure for patients waiting to be seen by a doctor, that all communication should be written at a 6th grade level to better the chances that all who read would comprehend the message.

Remember to avoid medical jargon and abbreviations that the person with whom you are speaking won't understand. As caregivers, we are used to speaking with other caregivers who understand the jargon. When choosing the right words caregivers should try to keep conversations with patients and their family's focused on the human being and not their illness. This focus allows a caregiver to focus on the right words and thus provide an empathetic communication exchange and avoid being seen as just clinical.

Paraverbal Communication

Paraverbal communication is the vocal part of speech. It's the tone of your voice, the volume at which you deliver the message, and the speed at which the sentence is spoken that tells a greater story than the actual words you are using. In other words, it's not what you say, it's how you say it.

If you are aware of the *tone* of your voice, you can begin to see how a simple inflection on a particular consonant or vowel can completely change the meaning of a sentence. That tone might convey a sense of condescension, sarcasm, or doubt. On the opposite side of the tone scale your tone may give a sense of happiness, excitement, or eager anticipation. Each of these vocal expressions can be applied to the words we're speaking and can convey a more effective message than the words themselves. I will give you an example of tone and how to use it to relay a message.

If you have ever had to raise a teenage girl, then surely you have been exposed to paraverbal communication. In my experience, during an argument with a teenager, they almost exclusively use nonverbal and paraverbal communication when speaking. For example, a teenager might say, "Dad, can I go to the mall?"

The parent might answer, "You can't go now. It's already ten pm!"

The teenager may give the rebuttal, "But, *daaaad* (hip shift, head tilt with an ascending volume on the words and a slow down for affect....oh forgot about the eyeball roll), everyone is going!" Message delivered. She doesn't like your decision.

Still not convinced? Try this little experiment. I want you to write down on a piece of paper the sentence: "I didn't call you stupid." Now take a moment to read the sentence aloud with a monotone voice, no tone, average volume, and a normal speed. What does the sentence say to you? That sentence is basically making a statement that the person saying it is simply stating that they didn't call you stupid. Now read the sentence again, only this time I want you to emphasize (use tone) the word "call." Now what does the sentence mean? What is the feeling you now get from the person saying it? If you are like most people, the sentence now sounds like the person who is saying it is being coy and saying I didn't *call* you stupid (but I thought it!). The word or verbal structure is the same, and yet the meaning is completely different. You can do this with each word in that sentence and each time the meaning, or feeling, changes to produce a different message.

The *volume* of your voice is the second component to paraverbal communication. The decibel level that you choose can tell the recipient that you are angry when you speak loudly or that you are in a peaceful state when you speak softly. How many times have you caught yourself speaking loudly to a patient when you see that based on physical appearance that they are "very old"? Isn't it a natural reaction to increase the volume of your voice? The belief is that we are being thoughtful and increasing the volume of our voice to make sure that the patient hears us, but in reality we are making an assumption based on physical appearance. Do you raise the volume of your voice when you enter a young patient's room? Unless there is some physical reason, most likely you don't.

The third component of paraverbal communication is pace or what some call cadence. We can use the speed at which we deliver the words to send a message. For example, let's say you are sitting down with a caregiver to discuss the reason for a pattern of tardiness. You set aside some time to discuss this issue so that the caregiver understands the consequences of their actions. Right before you start the conversation, you remember you have something that was due to the boss an hour ago. As your conversation begins, you're rushed, so you speak quickly, and after you've delivered your message, you quickly say, "Is there anything you want to discuss?" Is that caregiver likely to discuss their issues or have they already picked up on the speed at which you delivered the message and believe that you don't really want to hear their side of the story? Although this helps you get to that overdue report more quickly, it breaks down the relationship you have with the caregiver because they don't feel heard.

Barriers to Paraverbal Communication

There are obvious barriers when it comes to using tone effectively to communicate. Some are the same as our verbal barriers. For example, different cultures and ethnicities communicate with certain tones in their voices. These tones are more due to dialect than to attitude or emotion.

Personal emotions can certainly influence your paraverbal communication. Have you ever asked someone a question and they answered it with a sharp tone? "Wake up on the wrong side of the bed today?"

Of course there is also the title of this book, *No Time to Care*. Caregivers frequently tell me they feel like task doers hurrying from task to task to get each one done, rarely ever acknowledging the patient. Healthcare environments today are a natural barrier to paraverbal communication purely due to its fast paced nature and our inability to slow down and interact with our patients.

The final barrier is not related to sending messages, but rather receiving them. Making wrong assumptions can be detrimental when dealing with caregivers. There can be more than one message that is being relayed and based on how the person receives those paraverbal messages will determine the outcome. If you want a practical example that occurs daily you have to look no further than your cell phone. Text messaging removes all paraverbal and nonverbal cues from communication. We rely simply on the words that are on the screen to determine the meaning of the message. Have you ever sent a text message and the meaning of your message is completely missed? While a person writes a text they are mentally supplying the paraverbal and nonverbal communication in their head. However, when the message is sent to you through cyberspace the paraverbal and nonverbal communication stays behind. Only the words are sent. When that message reaches the intended recipient, they will read it and supply the nonverbal and paraverbal clues they imagine you attached to this message before sending it. This is very difficult to do since you are only left with the words to provide the actual message. This is why it is believed that paraverbal communication plays more of a role in effective communication than verbal.

Keys to Effective Paraverbal Communication

Understanding the important role of paraverbal communication is the first step. This means that we must evaluate our role in communication in a different way. What are your current emotions? Am I annoyed, and if so, then a greater regulation of those feelings is needed and the tone of my voice must be monitored. Are you in a rush giving someone his or her discharge instructions? If so, then you must be conscious of that and slow down your words when conversations warrant it. Perhaps talking slower is needed, but in order to make up time multitask whatever still needs to be done. According to an Agency for Healthcare Research and Quality (AHRQ), patients are 30 percent more likely to be readmitted if they don't understand their discharge instructions. Speaking to patients at a normal or slow speed, which helps them to understand, can reduce costs and, more importantly, provide patients with better care.[20]

Consider the volume of your voice. Suppose you're communicating to a grandmother who has custody of her granddaughter because her daughter is

---

[20] AHRQ. (2012). Project Red: Reengineering the discharge process. Retrieved May 2,2015 from https://cahps.ahrq.gov/surveys-guidance/hospital/hcahps_slide_sets/project_red/projectredtranscript.html

a heroin addict. She has brought her grandchild to the emergency department because the child has been sick for a week. You're not going to speak to the grandmother in a loud voice and say, "Hey, I just want to let you know that your granddaughter has leukemia!" That's not the way you would deliver that message. At that moment, a soft tone with low volume is appropriate to deliver that sensitive message. Use the volume of your voice to deliver the message in the delicate way it is intended to be delivered.

Nonverbal Communication

What It Is

Nonverbal communication can be simply thought of as "body language." It is the messages that we send to others through our gestures, our facial expressions and body posture. Making eye contact, leaning forward, or simply smiling all relay messages to those who receive them. These messages can be interpreted in different ways. With a tilt of the head and folding of the arms, you can transfer the meaning of your words from "I'm interested" to "I'm not even listening". We are constantly conveying nonverbal cues whether we realize it or not. The recognition of these behaviors start at a young age. Emotional Comprehension Development happens early in life. Researchers (Bullock & Russell, 1985; Cutting & Dunn, 1999) have found that children as young as 4 and 5 years old are able to recognize and name the facial expressions of basic emotions when presented in pictures. Nonverbal communication plays a strong role in communication and the development of this skill occurs early in life.[21]

Barriers to Nonverbal Communication

Your nonverbal messages are constantly out in front of you. Others can read them, and if not aware of what those clues are saying about you, then you are destined to send either mixed messages or just bad ones. I tell caregivers all the time that when they walk into a patient's room and go to Bed B, but pass Bed A without acknowledging the person in that bed, then they're sending a nonverbal message that "You're not as important to me." It may not be your intention. You may be focused on the task at hand, but that lack of acknowledgment can make a patient or family member feel like you are cold and uncaring. These are easy opportunities to use nonverbal

---

[21] Russel, J. A., & Bullock, M. (1986). On the dimensions preschoolers use to interpret facial expressions of emotion. Developmental Psychology, 22, 97-102.

communication, like a smile or a hand wave, to relay your acknowledgment of the human being laying in that bed.

Think about the power of nonverbal communication. I tell people all the time that your nonverbal communication will be judged long before you ever say a word. Not convinced? The next time you are walking down the hall be cognizant of the distance at which you make a determination as to whether you are going to say hello to the person walking toward you from the opposite direction. Was it 5 feet? 10 feet? 20 feet? When did they make the decision to acknowledge you? There are of course many factors that influence each person's behavior. You make a judgment based on that person's body language and physical appearance. Perhaps it depends on your own mood and emotional state. The perception of your behavior by others can be seen as a barrier that you have no control over. By just having an awareness of this issue, you can help control its affect.

There are other barriers to consider. Cultural and physical barriers may create an obstacle. Blindness would be an obvious physical issue. From a cultural perspective some cultures believe making eye contact is not encouraged or speaking directly to a woman is not allowed. If not understood, this behavior could send the wrong nonverbal messages.

Sending the wrong nonverbal message can be felt when the person you are interacting with is distracted or is continuously interrupted. Facebook, Instagram and other social media apps are the enemies of nonverbal communication. Constantly distracted by our phones, we can be seen as uncaring and disinterested when these apps distract us. Acknowledging this potential barrier, I always prepare for any conversation that I need to have one on one with caregivers by silencing my cell phone, turning the computer screen off, and asking my assistant to answer my calls.

Keys to Effective Nonverbal Communication

As leaders, it's important that we recognized nonverbal cues, both in the people we are communicating with as well as our own. Once recognized, we can master these skills, send the messages we want to send, and avoid the ones that were unintended. Effective communication can only occur when the nonverbal matches the verbal. If it does not, there can be confusion, frustration, and even anger.

For instance, I remember working with a leader who came to me one day very frustrated because people in her department did not seem to feel comfortable coming to her to share hot topics or valuable gossip about issues affecting the care of the patients. I don't believe in encouraging malicious gossip, but knowing the hot topics, or what's going on in the unit, does have its merit. "Why do you think that is?" she asked. I didn't know, but I asked her to let me know the next time she had a conversation. I asked that she try to have it in the Trauma Room where I could observe her through the glass doors to see if I could determine why there was a lack of trust.

A few days later she found that opportunity. I observed her for about 10 minutes. A colleague asked if he could speak to her in private and so she took him into the trauma room and closed the door. As I observed the interaction, I noticed a particular nonverbal behavior. During her conversation, this leader was standing with her arms folded across her chest. Later when I had a chance to talk to her, I asked, "How did you think that went?"

She said, "I don't know. He seemed pretty frustrated and I don't feel I really got through to him." I asked her what the conversation had been about, and she told me that he had shared an idea about how the trauma rooms might be reorganized. "What were your thoughts?" I asked.

"I told him I would ask the Best Practice committee to look into it." She replied.

Ah. "I know what your problem is. The entire time you were talking your arms were folded, your head was tilted, and the hips were shifted to the right relaying the message 'You're wasting your breath'."

"No, I wasn't!" she said.

"Yes," I nodded. "You were. So, basically, what you were telling him verbally was yes, I understand and hear what you're saying, but nonverbally you were saying 'nope, that's a dumb idea.'"

So, I told her, "We're going to get you a gift." The next day, I brought her a lab coat, and I suggested that every time she had a conversation with someone, she should consciously put her hands into the pockets of her jacket. I told her to think of those pockets as magnets and that her hands were made of metal. She did as I suggested, and it wasn't long before she began to notice a difference in how others were responding to her.

Nonverbal behaviors can be as easy as sitting down. I preach to physicians all the time to sit when giving discharge instructions. Why? Because it conveys to the patient that you have the time and want to make sure they truly understand their discharge instructions. I challenge you. Do this experiment. Discharge 3 people and sit to give the instructions. When you do this you only have 1 minute or less to give the instructions. Then discharge your next 3 patients but stay standing by the door as you do it. Take as much time as you want. Then have someone survey the patients before they leave about how they felt about the caregiver providing the discharge instructions. I guarantee the first group will be more satisfied than the second simply because the caregiver sat down to give the instructions. We call it our "Commit to Sit" program.

We can't underestimate the impact that nonverbal communication has on how we are perceived by others. It can be difficult, though, to recognize the nonverbal messages we may be inadvertently sending. Did you know that you roll your eyes when someone tells you something that you don't agree with? You probably don't. But isn't it important to know this so that you can filter your reactions in order for staff to believe that you are interested in what they are telling you? That takes practice. Be brave and ask for a third party perspective and assessment from someone you trust—a manager, friend or colleague. Then practice what you are not good at and you will become the type of leader that others want to communicate with.

COMMUNICATING TO STAFF

Effective communication is essential at all levels of leadership—whether communicating with staff or communicating to them. It's not only vital to being a great leader, but is relative in terms of supporting those around you. The majority of our day consists of either sending messages or receiving them. This is why as a leader we must first learn effective ways to communicate with and then find ways to provide the communication necessary to help caregivers feel engaged in the process.

In the absence of information, caregivers tend to fill in the blanks; they'll make up their own stories. They will take whatever they hear, whether rumors or speculations, and make it their reality. Perception is reality and that perceived reality can be devastating for the culture you're trying to build.

Since you understand that those who are informed are far less likely to speculate or start rumors, what are your steps as a leader to ensure that they are well informed and are given chances to ask questions? There are a wide range of ways that you can communicate with your staff and you should employ all of them: in person and face-to-face, through email, through meetings and, more and more commonly, through a wide array of social media options.

What type of communication you use depends on whom your audience is that you are communicating with at the time. If you want to connect with a group of leaders, then perhaps a written communication plan is needed so that you may keep track of the information or ideas discussed. If you are communicating with the caregivers who fall into the millennials generation, then social media is a form of communication they are used to using so capitalizing on that will increase your chances of them receiving the information.

In my many years of leadership, I have witnessed that leaders rely solely on a monthly staff meeting to communicate with staff. The negative to monthly staff meetings is that caregivers must wait an entire month to receive additional communication. Another issue is ensuring that all caregivers are receiving the messages. Have you ever been to a staff meeting where every caregiver from the unit was in attendance? Of course you haven't. If someone misses the staff meeting, now what? Do they just go a month without receiving the information? Perhaps you are relying on them, in their spare time, to read the minutes and then ask questions? Staff meetings can be helpful, but they should be just one part of the communication process.

Communication should be a consistent process that happens throughout the day, throughout the week, and throughout the month. How long after you leave a meeting do you start to forget what was said? Information is short lived unless it is repeated and reinforced. There are many ways to have that communication and in turn help caregivers receive and remember the information you are providing.

In this busy healthcare world there are lots of things to remember so information retention is often poor. My old boss would always say to me that it takes mentioning something 7 times before a thought moves from their short-term memory to their long term memory. Providing multiple reminders will help increase retention of information. Some of the following ideas below have been used to provide information in different ways in order to make an impact.

Hot Topics

When it comes to communication you can provide it, you can receive it, or you can seek it out. Identifying the hot topics affecting the unit morale is very important. A leader needs to get really good at the practice of seeking out information in order to prevent issues from getting worse or being proactive to prevent a negative outcome. To begin to understand the hot topics in the department a leader should ask themselves, and for that matter others—what are the caregivers talking about? Maybe it's that people are upset that a policy was put in place without their input or that the techs are really angry at the nurses because a nurse called a tech lazy. It doesn't matter what the issue is, the fact that it's causing disharmony on the unit is what needs to be brought to your attention. If you're unaware of these issues, you will not be able to address them, and the conflict will continue.

Let's be real. You can't be present all the time or aware of all the issues affecting the department. This is why relationship building with your caregivers is imperative to building a culture where caregivers want the department to succeed because they are invested. This vested interest often creates a "not on my watch" attitude. It may not happen right away, but eventually the caregivers will start holding each other accountable. Engaged caregivers want to express their concerns and inform you of the issues that are affecting the department. If you build the right relationships, they will find ways to get you the information you need to be on top of the hot topics.

Huddles or Huggles

Huggles provide an opportunity for you to check in with staff on a daily basis and provide them with real time information that affect the caregivers' working environment. The reason we call them huggles is simple. Caregivers complained that our shift huddles are often only focused on information, statistics, and metrics goals. They understood the information was necessary, but wanted to find a way to make these important meetings more positive. They wanted to find a way to instill some positive energy into the beginning of the shift. So, the huggle was created.

Our huggles are held every day at various times, which are based on the arrival patterns of our caregivers. We start our first huggle of the day at 9am, then repeat it at 11am when more caregivers arrive and then again at 7pm for the night shift. These times are what is best for our particular schedule, but it may vary for your department. They are very simple and designed to be no longer than five minutes. We begin with the immediate news of the day. This usually consists of what staffing looks like, and if there are any callouts, and then we discuss any new policy or procedures that caregivers may have questions about. We then ask if there are any rumors that need to be dispelled. For a few years, this is where the huggle ended until staff started to comment that they didn't look forward to these brief meetings because it was only filled with tasks that they needed to do or reminders that they weren't doing. Their feelings were that they always ended with negativity.

The Colleague Engagement Committee (or what we like to refer to as the fun committee) was asked to find a way to end the huddles on a positive note. The simple answer: end every huddle with a positive comment or story. They wanted to assign one person per huggle to end the gathering with a creative and positive story, comment, or idea.

At first, the caregivers didn't really want to be a part of these huggles. They wanted positivity but they didn't want to be the ones responsible for creating it. This is where accountability comes into play. Once again the caregivers saw the value in the idea because it was generated by their peers, not leadership. Holding others accountable is much easier when the rules of the many outweigh the feelings of a few.

It was a little rough at first. There would be caregivers that were assigned the positivity ending who got in front of the group and said, "It's going to be a sunny day outside." After a few of those, we made a decision that anyone that didn't put forth their best effort had to come up with a new positivity message at the next huggle, and then the next huggle, and the next until they showed a positive effort. People quickly got it right the first time.

It was great to watch. People kept trying to be better than the last huggler. It became a bit of a competition. One person sang a little song. The next made a funny poem. Creativity started to emerge. One of my favorites was the creation of ER bingo. At the end of the huddle, staff members were given a card. The card mimicked a bingo card, but instead of numbers filling the squares, there were tasks and achievements that filled each square. Some examples were, "I got pooped on", "I saved a life", or "I started my 15th IV." The concept was the same: fill the box in the pattern designated for the game and you win a prize. How awesome is that!

Even the leadership team got into the creativity act. I remember one of our clinical leads told a story about her auto mechanic. I remember thinking where is this story going? She talked about the wonderful service that they provided and then reminded everyone about the power of exceeding expectations in this business we call healthcare. They're using my quotes. I love it!

Another huggle that stands out in my mind was done by one of our ER techs. She told everyone a story about how she had brought her mother into the emergency department over the weekend. She stated that she saw the care her mother received from a different set of eyes. She then told everyone that she was proud to be a part of such a caring and compassionate team. I remember the slight pause and silence that filled the room as we waited for her next statement. She then stood in the middle of the room and said, "So, since you all provided such wonderful care to my mother, I would like to give you all a kiss!" It was at this point that she reached behind the desk and pulled out a little basket filled with Hershey's Kisses.

Game Plan Tip: Huggle Cards

When communicating to staff it is important that everyone on the leadership team be on the same page. Consistent messaging is necessary to create an open communication environment and show consistency among leaders. Our leadership team always meets the first Thursday of every month. It is during this meeting that we discuss, among other things, the different information that we need to disseminate to the caregivers. Our problem, however, was that once we all left the meeting, leaders would forget what we needed to relay, information provided was inconsistent and made the leadership team look unorganized. In order to maintain consistency and ensure all caregivers were getting the same message we created the Huggle card.

Step 1: At the beginning of the leadership meeting, distribute 5 x 8 cards to all of the clinical leaders. The clinical leads are the ones that run the huggles for all shifts. Some would refer to this group as assistant nurse managers or permanent charge nurses.

Step 2: As the leadership team discusses issues that affect the department, identify issues that are huggle-worthy. This allows each leader on the team to have the same huggle topics, in the same order, so that they can, in turn, share them with their teams during huggles.

It's important to ensure that communication is consistent and our 5 x 8 cards are just one way of doing this. There's nothing more damaging than leaders sending two different messages about the same topic. Sometimes the cards are filled with 10 or more topics. The idea is not to talk about them all at once. The first week we will discuss the first three on the list. The next week, three new huggle card topics. Messages are consistent, timely, and strategic.

Town Hall Meetings

Town hall meetings are different than staff meetings. At our town hall meetings, the only person in a leadership position that attends is me. I sit down with the staff and I say, "Let's just have an open meeting. This is your time. I have no agenda. I'm just here so we can talk about things that are bothering you—things that you think we can improve on, answer questions, dispel rumors or anything else you want to talk about."

It can take a while in town halls for people to feel comfortable to speak freely. Even after the tenth meeting, where the open format is well known, that lingering hesitation is always present at the beginning of the meeting. People are often hesitant to talk, but usually one person will be brave. They will raise their hand and ask the first question and the rest of the staff will watch your reaction to the question closely. It is imperative that you take no question personally! A quick response filled with emotion will stifle the energy and create even more hesitation.

You have to prepare mentally for the meeting. Expect some negativity. Expect that they may be passionate about a certain topic, and that they may jump right out of the gate with "I hate it when..." Focus on removing the emotion from every question and, more importantly, be open to their ideas and try to find value in every comment that is made.

Although freedom of speech is encouraged, there are two rules for these discussions that we always follow:

1. We can speak about an individual who is not in the room; however, it must be done with respect and be followed by opportunities for improvement that can be offered to that person. In other words, you can't just complain without offering suggestions for improvement.
2. This leads to the second rule. If you have an issue with something, state it, but somewhere in your statement better be a suggestion for improvement or at least an acknowledgement that you don't know how to fix it.

After each meeting, I document the issues identified and the ideas presented on a piece of paper. There are 3 columns. The first column states what the problem is, the idea to be implemented, or the roadblock to be removed. We call this the "What" column. The second column is called the "Who" column. It identifies who is going to gather additional information or implement the plan. And finally, the third column is referred to as the "By When" column. This is where the desired completion date for the project is noted.

Many great ideas have come out of these town halls. We prioritize the list into three categories. The first group is the low-hanging fruit items. The second group is the "council worthy" items. And the final list is the "these are going be really hard to change." Again, this is honest and open communication where the vulnerable leader is admitting that they may not be able to fix some things the staff considers to be broken. The list is then posted for all to see. Caregivers are asked to look at the list and provide feedback and suggestions if possible. As each issue is addressed and fixed, they are crossed out with a highlighter and the solution is posted so that the feedback loop is closed.

Leadership Feedback

In addition to rumor control, working barriers identified, and general questions, I also welcome feedback about the leadership team. That's right, I openly solicited feedback about the leadership team. We call it opportunities for improvement (OPIs). I promise the leadership team that I will ensure that all feedback is constructive and something they could use to make themselves better. In turn I remind the staff that any feedback provided must be constructive in nature and be void of negative sentiments. That trust amongst caregivers took a little bit of time to develop, but it only takes a few mentions without repercussions to give the caregivers a sense that it is safe to speak up.

This process was uncomfortable at first for my leadership team. I heard things like "It's not fair that he's listening to their issues without me being present," and "Why can't they just say it to me?" Well, let's think about that. How easy is it for you to confront your leader in a positive and constructive way? How easy is it for a leader to be open to receiving criticism from the caregivers they lead? The reality is that if there is no forum for open discussion, then issues and problems will fester under the radar until they become too big. They usually manifest themselves by caregivers acting out or creating a negative working environment. Leadership, including me, needs to always be open to feedback. The caregivers, however, need to be sure that they provide feedback that is constructive and always offers suggestion for improvement. If it is not presented in that way, the topic is closed and we move to the next topic.

As mentioned, my leadership team is not the only group who is available for OPIs. Caregivers also have the freedom to tell me what they think of a new program or policy or perhaps about my own style of leadership. Again, what good is the criticism if no one hears it or uses it to make change for the better? My door is always open and caregivers are encouraged to come speak to me one on one. It's my job to create an environment where the caregivers feel comfortable having those conversations. Of course, this takes time and trust. Once built, this two-way open communication can be healthy and beneficial.

Hearing constructive feedback and being open to hearing constructive feedback are two separate things. Being open to it is where leaders separate themselves. However, this is a skill that takes practice. How you receive it is important. A leader must be aware of their nonverbal communication when someone gives them feedback. If you fold your arms or roll your eyes, then the immediate feeling is that you are not open to hearing what they are saying and no one will ever offer you feedback ever again.

The second key to receiving criticism is creating a working environment where everyone knows that mistakes will happen. I always like to do this by reminding caregivers that it is our response to those mistakes that makes the difference. If you make a mistake, admit it and then apologize. By not admitting your mistakes, you give the impression that you are perfect, which can lead to unrealistic expectations from your staff. The more real that you can be, not only as a leader, but as a human being, the more likely caregivers will follow that standard. Some criticism is deserved and appreciated. Appreciated by you and more importantly appreciated by them.

People issues do not make it to the list Who, What, By When list. That feedback is provided to the person privately and directly. Remember, the focus of these meetings should be nonjudgmental suggestions that will be use to educate and help the team grow and never be used as a punishment.

In leadership there are some skills that, if added, can make you a better leader and there are other skills that are absolutely imperative that you have. These skills take time to learn and even more time to perfect. Effective communication with and to staff builds the trust needed to have a cohesive team. If staff feel valued and heard, they are more likely to go out of their way to positively contribute to the unit. Effective communication is needed in today's frenzied healthcare environment by both leaders and the caregivers who rely on them for guidance.

CHAPTER 5
POWER OF THE PEOPLE

In previous chapters, we talked about the importance of motivation, effective communication, and getting everybody on the same page, all sharing the same vision—a vision that they helped to create. The Clinical Excellence Commitment Board is a critical beginning step here, but more is needed if you want to ensure caregiver engagement. Once a common vision and expectations have been established, documented, and committed to, the next step is to sustain these behaviors.

That's not an easy thing to do. It takes ongoing effort and focus. Anytime you create change, you also create anxiety. Too often, employees view new patient or caregiver engagement initiatives as the "flavor of the month" because many caregivers have seen these programs come and go. They are sustained for a period of time and then the program or energy around the imitative fades away because focus is lost. It takes leadership persistence and caregiver patience to work beyond the period of time where programs convert from a daily task to true culture change.

EMPOWERING THE CAREGIVERS

What is true empowerment? Some leaders think that to empower others all they need to do is give the caregivers an idea and then let them figure out a way to get the desired result. Empowerment isn't something you *do* to others, it's really more about what you don't do. It's more about getting out of their way and having the courage to let things happen. Empowerment is reinforced when you allow caregivers to try new ideas, and when you encourage them to learn from any mistakes made and use that experience to create an even better plan.

Empowerment can only happen when you, as a leader, feel confident that the group making the decisions respects and understands the vision of the department. Without a clear vision, how is a group expected to make decisions that will foster the culture that you are trying to develop? When the caregivers are empowered, they feel in control of their jobs, themselves, and their success. Laschinger, Almost, & Tuer-Hodes (2003) studied the characteristics of empowered nurses who work in Magnet hospitals. They noted when nurses feel empowered, they:

➢ Have a greater sense of autonomy
➢ Have better physician relationships
➢ Have control over their practice environment[22]

To support an independent free-thinking department where the caregivers are empowered, leaders must provide the needed environment that encourages people to work together and supports the creative thinking process. Leaders must be brave enough to let go of their control. That is difficult for some. As a leader, you are responsible for the overall care that is provided within that unit. It takes courage to truly put that care in the hands of the caregivers by empowering them to make decisions that affect the patient experience.

So, how does a leader reduce their anxiety level when relinquishing control? Simple—provide the structure that caregivers can use to make those decisions. That does not mean create rules to follow. It means that you are providing them with guidance to help them make those decisions that are the best for caregivers and patients and their families. There are two basic questions that all caregivers are required to ask themselves before they make an independent free-thinking decision in our department.

1. "Is the decision we are about to make the right thing for the patient and their family?
2. "Is this going to cost a lot of money?"

---

[22] Spence-Laschinger, H. K., Almost, J., Tuer-Hodes, D., (2003). Workplace empowerment and magnet hospital characteristics making the link. JONA, 33(7/8), 410-422.

If the answer is "yes," then "no," go for it. If the answer is "yes" and "yes," then I need to be consulted for approval. Even when the committee "goes for it," the group stills runs the idea by me, not because they have to, because they want to. They value my opinion, not because they feel obligated or are required, but because they see me as a valuable member of the team.

Whatever the decision, if it turns out to be a mistake, then learn from it and come back better the next time. I believe that some of the greatest lessons I have learned as a leader, and for that matter, as a human being, have come from the mistakes I have made in my life. I believe the same applies to the caregivers.

If a mistake is made by a caregiver, how you react to that mistake is key. As a leader, you must be prepared to hear the truth. If your verbal or nonverbal reaction to the news that a mistake has been is made is anything but understanding and calm, the caregivers will hesitate to risk coming forward in the future. This takes practice. You must regulate your response using nonverbal and paraverbal skills, which we covered in the previous chapter (see Chapter 4).

Allow People to be Brave

When do you know as a leader that the culture that you have worked so hard to achieve is now a permanent fixture of the work environment? How do you know that the caregivers are engaged in ensuring that the care they provide creates the best possible experience for patients and their families? Always looking for the tangible, leaders seek definitive signs that they have finally achieved success. The answers to these questions are not easily answered. It is not a black and white situation. There are, however, telltale signs that part, if not all, of the culture has taken shape. For example, when employees make decisions based on what's right for the patient and not whether or not the consequences of their actions may be punishable in the court of leadership opinion, it is a good sign. When that fear of retribution is removed, caregivers will start to advocate for patients in a way that creates a more focused patient experience. They will take chances when they believe it is the right thing to do for the patients. They will be proactive in seeking out new ways to transform the patient experience.

Let me give you an example of when I started to realize that all of our hard work was starting to pay off. When a patient comes into our ER with chest pain, we have a rule that within 5 minutes, the patient gets an EKG.

One day, one of our ER techs was sitting in the ER triage area when a patient came in with chest pain. The tech performed the EKG soon after the triage nurse ordered it. About a half hour later, the patient, whose EKG had been read as negative by the ER physician, was still sitting in the waiting room. Another very sick patient, had arrived and the triage nurse had taken the patient immediately back to a room to be treated.

As the ER tech stood watch over the waiting room patients, she noticed that the patient that she had performed an EKG on just 30 minutes prior "Didn't look too good." She approached the patient and asked if he was okay. He said he was feeling "a little weird" and he thought his chest pain was coming back. The question she asked herself was, *Gee, should I do another EKG?* This is despite knowing that doing a repeat EKG requires an order from a physician. All the other caregivers were busy caring for patients. Alone and not knowing what additional options she might have, this tech made a conscious decision based on the two questions we always ask ourselves in our department.

Is this the right thing to do for the patient? The answer was clearly yes.

If I do this repeat EKG, will it cost a lot of money? The answer was clearly no.

She repeated the EKG without an order, and she showed it to the doctor. The patient's EKG showed he was now having a heart attack. She called the charge nurse, and said, "I need to bring this patient back now." No one questioned her; they brought him to a room and they saved his life. Without a culture that encourages free-thinking and risk-taking, this caregiver may have simply followed the rules. Without fear of reprimand, she did something that was clearly against policy, but did so after asking the two fundamental questions.

Make a mistake. That's fine. We'll learn from it, and we'll be better next time. This culture helped create strong relationships between caregivers and leaders. This strong engagement helped this caregiver feel empowered to do what she thought was right and to save a man's life. It ultimately led to a patient experience the caregiver, and patient for that matter, will never forget.

Relinquishing Power

How do you respond when caregivers come to you with an idea that they want to implement, but you believe that it will not be successful? Giving permission to a group to try a new idea or implement a new process that they came up with can instill confidence in those caregivers and show them that their opinions are truly valued. I help young leaders all the time understand that sometimes it is worth allowing others to try, and to fail, and to use it as a learning opportunity to improve. Instead of thinking "that's not going to work because…" Try to force yourself to think instead, *Why not, why shouldn't I let them try this?*

If you can't fight the urge to insist that their way is wrong and that they should try yours, then they will begin to doubt their ability to make a difference. "Why should we suggest new things if they always get shot down?" Too many of those reactions, and you will never get another suggestion again. In reality, as a leader, some of your initial response is still your lingering inability to let go, mixed with the belief that what is being presented to you will never work. The truth is even in failure there is success. Allow the caregivers to try, then fail, and they will find a way to make it right while appreciating your willingness to be open to their ideas.

Is it going to cost a lot of money? Some people cringe at that second question. Caring for people should not be about the money! That, however, is the reality of doing business and, remember, healthcare is big business. We have to be concerned about the costs of the things that we do. That's just the way it is. But, freethinking ideas do not need to cost a lot of money.

Here's an example. An ER tech was walking by a room where a woman was sitting at the bedside of her husband, and she happened to hear the woman crying. She investigated and found out that it was the couple's 60th wedding anniversary, and the woman was sad to be spending it in the hospital. "I'm so sorry to hear that," the tech said, and consoled the woman. She left the room and tried to find the charge nurse, but she couldn't locate her. Without asking for permission, she opened the service recovery box, which was only to be used to recover dissatisfied patients or families, and took a cafeteria gift certificate from the box.

This caregiver told me after the fact that she was worried she would get in trouble because she knows senior administration monitors that box to ensure no one is stealing from it. She also knew, though, that the culture in our Emergency Department was to find ways to create a great experience for our patients and their families, even if that meant taking a risk.

She used the certificate to buy some Twinkies, opened them up, put them on a paper plate in a circle like they were a cake and took two straws and stuck them in the Twinkie cake as if they were candles. She then grabbed a unit clerk and a physician and together they went back to the couple in the room where she said, "I hope you don't mind. We did something special for you. We'd like to sing happy anniversary to you." And that's what they did—over the top of a Twinkie cake with straws for candles.

They made the woman cry again. But this time it was tears of appreciation and happiness. It didn't take a lot of time, effort, or money to create that joy. It simply took an empowered caregiver and a creative mind to take a chance. Sometimes we have a tendency to think that patient engagement requires expensive programs and a lot of money. That's not necessarily true. Sometimes it's the little things that can create the greatest impact. When caregivers are not afraid to do what is right for the patients, creative restraint is lifted, and, in my experience, caregivers come up with some pretty awesome ideas.

In this case, the woman was so moved she wrote six letters—one to the CEO, one to the COO, one to me, two to the local papers, and one to the Chief Nursing Officer. That was a lot of impact for a seemingly small gesture. The patient was touched, and the staff was proud of the experience they were able to give this woman.

SELF-GOVERNANCE: WE THE PEOPLE!

Many organizations say they have a self-governing department, but, in reality, it is used simply as a vehicle to achieve goals set forth by administration. There is a distinct difference between telling someone your plan and asking them to get it done as opposed to identifying a problem, asking the group to find a solution, and then figuring out a way to implement it. The latter not only gives the caregivers a say in what the change will be, but it also allows them to control it. This is vital when it comes to change. The more vested they are, the more likely they are to adopt the change. The power to truly implement self-governance also starts again with a leader's ability to relinquish control and to allow caregivers to make decisions that will affect the flow of the department.

Self-governance is achieved through the development of shared commitments and the opportunity to be accountable for the success of the department. Caregivers will be more engaged in programs they themselves have created. They implement them more quickly and will monitor them more closely to ensure success. With engaged caregivers the focus is shifted to reward those who positively contribute to the success of the department.

These engaged caregivers are also more willing to stand up to other colleagues who are negative and not vested, and hold them accountable.

Self-governance That Works

There are many self-governing structures that work. It's not a new concept, but it's one that can be daunting to establish and then make sustainable. Our self-governance model is based on the idea that if you want something (in this case the ability to make decisions that impact you), you need to be willing to give something in return. True empowerment demands both of these requirements. In our case, what the caregivers need to give is their time.

Each caregiver must sign up for a committee; it is a requirement of the Clinical Excellence Commitment Standards. This includes all caregivers, from nurses to unit clerks to techs to physicians. Yes, I said physicians! It's an expectation for all.

Like in any program or culture change, there is a need to find a way to keep it fresh and fun for everyone. Engagement in the process will wane if the tasks at hand are seen as mundane and uninspiring. Naturally, the excitement of these committees will begin to wear off over time, so how do you keep people engaged in this worthwhile process? How do you help caregivers believe that there is value in attending the meeting and that they have a part in building the culture? I call it excuse busting. There are many excuses people will give as to why they cannot attend the meetings.

"It's too far to drive."

"I have no one to watch my kids."

"The times don't work for me."

I've heard them all. As I see it, we have two paths as leaders that we can take. The first is the "hit them over the head and demand attendance, or we will punish you" approach. Personal experience has shown that this method is ineffective. The caregivers will rebel on purpose and also recruit others to rebel as well. The second is the excuse busting approach, where we either anticipate the excuses before they occur or address them as they come up to find solutions for the caregivers to be successful.

Game Plan Tip: Excuse Busting

Having poor attendance when we first started our shared governance committees, we pulled the Best Practice committee together to determine what we needed to do to help other caregivers be successful (The best practice committee seemed to have the best attendance). There were many reasons cited for not being able to attend, so I challenged the committee to find ways to defeat the excuses. The solutions were as follows.

➢ Each committee would pick the day of the week that they would meet. No two committees were permitted to have the same day. This helped stop the "I can't meet on Mondays because that's when I get my dog groomed" excuse. If you are on the Best Practice committee and they meet on Mondays, a day that you are unavailable, then pick a different committee that meets on a day that you are available.

➢ Each group will have alternating times when they meet. For example, the January meeting will occur at 7am and the February meeting will occur at 6pm. With alternating times, this limits the excuse "I have to get my children on the bus in the morning, so I can't make the meetings." Okay, no problem, then perhaps the 7am meetings are not for you, but now you can make the 6pm one. Again, lots of variety allows for more attendance flexibility.

➢ All meeting times and dates are posted a year in advance for all to see. Gone are the excuses "I can't attend because I work that day." Well, you work that day because you didn't pay attention to your meeting schedule. That puts the accountability back on the caregiver.

➢ "I've tried everything that I can, but I have small kids, so I can't drive in on my day off to attend meetings." No problem. Got you covered. We have a call-in line that you can use and attend the meeting from the comfort of your home, active participation of course is required.

I know what you are thinking. "If you give the call-in option, then caregivers will just call in and then put the phone on mute while they do the dishes. This is definitely a possibility, but we are smarter than that. As part of our committee chairperson training, we make sure that they focus not only on the people physically in attendance but also those on the phone. This requires a roll call so you know who is on the call and that they were there from beginning to end. The chairperson also randomly asks those on the phone for their opinion or solicits their feedback. I will be honest. In the beginning, we had a lot of conversations with attendees on the phone like the following "Hi there, Lisa, you've been a little quiet on the phone during this meeting, just wondering what your thoughts are on this new program we want to start?" *Silence.* Most likely Lisa was rushing to get the mute button off and frantically trying to come up with something to say, usually coming out with something like, "Yes, I'm here. I like the idea of the new program."

Great, Lisa. "What part do you like the most?" Again, silence.

"Um, I like it all?"

The chairperson would respond, "You have no idea what we were talking about, do you?" Silence, yet again. "Thank you for calling in, Lisa, but you can hang up now. You will not be getting credit for today's meeting." It only takes one or two of those conversations to occur before they get the picture. Calling from home is a not a free ride.

Merit-based Evaluations

Caregiver participation is the expectation. Members are expected to attend 50 percent of their committee meetings, and that expectation is set as a goal on their evaluation. Their ability to achieve these goals will directly impact their evaluation and, of course, their overall scores which can affect their raise. It becomes more real for any caregiver when you connect an expectation to their pocketbook. How so? Because we ensure that we truly reward people for their effort. The more you extend yourself beyond the expectation the better your score, the better the score, the bigger the raise.

Caregivers need to understand the importance of exceeding expectations and the value that brings to their pocketbook. For those who are extrinsically motivated, this is easy to understand. Receiving more money for the job that you do is welcomed by most people. Understanding that the effort that you put into making a patient's healthcare experience exceptional should be rewarded. Making this connection needs to be explicit. We accomplish this by truly providing merit-based raises. We have an evaluation process where there are four sections to the evaluation and each section is worth 25 percent in terms of contributing to the final salary, or "raise" calculation. Let's say one of those sections has five goals and one of those goals is coming to 50 percent of the meetings. If you don't make that goal, that's 20 percent off on the section that is worth 25 percent. Not meeting these goals can add up pretty quickly. This is just another way to make the connection between responsibility and accountability.

After all the evaluation scores are in, there is an adjustment period. We take all the scores and put them in ascending order. For those caregivers that failed to get a 2.0 or greater (means the caregiver at least met expectations), the raise money that was slated to them gets put back into the pot and then redistributed to those at the top of the list. If the average raise at the hospital is 2 percent, after redistributing the money, those who sit at the top of the list, or the top performers, will get a bigger raise. Perhaps it would be 2.5 percent or could be as high as 5 percent. Bottom line is that this method is a true pay for performance. The more you contribute, the more you make.

Not Everyone Wants to Govern

Of course, not all employees are going to leap at the chance to self-govern, to serve on a committee or, even worse, to chair or co-chair a committee. Leaders need to have some tricks up their sleeves to sometimes help nudge employees along. Here are a couple of tricks that I use quite successfully.

Musical Chairs

Remember that game you played as a child, musical chairs, where there would be 1 less chair than the number of people participating and everyone would walk around and around in a circle while music played? When the music stopped, everyone had to claim a chair. This program is similar. It's a way to reward people who show up or who follow the rules, and provide a disincentive for those who don't.

When you create committees, you create a specific number of spots on each committee based on how many employees you have. So, if you have four committees and 40 employees, you'll have 10 spots available on each committee and your sign-up sheets should reflect that with 10 spaces. Remember that all committees should have an equal number of representatives from the various disciplines that work on the unit. This includes nurses as well as techs, unit clerks, physicians, and anyone else that is considered part of your team.

In our case, we asked the caregivers to sign up for a committee during the Clinical Excellence Commitment Board signing party. This is a celebration where you sign the commitment board and then sign up for your committee. Of course, you need a pizza party to help energize the meeting (how much pizza have you eaten as a healthcare provider?). However, some caregivers don't come to the party for various reasons— some are legitimate while others just refuse to buy into the culture change you are trying to create. What happens to those caregivers? They get whatever committee is left. Once the 10 spots for a committee are filled, that committee is considered closed. Again, this is a reward for those that are engaged in the process, come to the meeting with eager anticipation, and want to be champions for the change. If you are first to sign up for a committee, then you will most likely join the committee of your choice. If you are not committed to change and blow off the meeting, then you will be assigned the committee with open spots.

An Old Wedding DJ Trick

Here's another way to encourage participation and "volunteerism." After you form a committee, the next step is to appoint a chair and co-chair. You might start by asking for volunteers. Of course, it is always nice to have a willing chairperson. If someone does volunteer to be chair, it is usually a caregiver who wants to do leadership in the future, so this is a great way to mentor and coach the future leaders of your department.

However, volunteers are rare, and the real challenge is finding a person who is willing to give it a shot. Hands do not usually fly up into the air, forcing you to choose among dozens of people, all dying for the chance to be a committee chairperson. If your staff is like mine, dead silence fills the room. People start to look at their watches, take the opportunity to check their cell phones, or some may even fake a cramp. Anything to avoid being selected.

So, here's what I do to make the chairperson selection process as fair as possible. I used to use this party trick when I worked as a DJ at weddings. Some of the biggest fights I have ever witnessed post-reception occurred over who got to take home the centerpieces! Seriously. So, before the wedding started, I would go through the room and tape a penny under one chair at the table. At the end of the night, I would tell everyone to feel under their chair and the one who found the penny got the centerpiece. The same concept applies here. Only this time, I taped one penny and one nickel under separate chairs. If volunteers come forward, that's great, but if no volunteers come forward, I say, "Okay, if there are no volunteers then I need everyone to stand up. I'm going to have you all flip your chairs over and look under your seat. The person with the nickel is the chair, and the person with the penny is the co-chair." This random approach means it is possible that a unit clerk could be chair and a nurse a co-chair. How perfect. Again, this helps support our culture that everyone is treated with respect regardless of their job title. What a great way to break down silos.

This is also a positive for caregivers who feel undervalued simply because of their job title. When a unit clerk is empowered to run a committee of her colleagues, she is seen as someone more than "the unit clerk," she is seen as the chairperson for the best practice committee. I've seen unit clerks move into tech positions, and then out of tech positions into nursing positions. Why? Because someone empowered them to feel valued as a team member. They are seen as equal participants in the overall culture, which ultimately builds self-confidence.

Coach Those Chairpeople

You have established your committees. People have signed up. You have your chairperson, so you are all set, nothing more to do. Right? Unfortunately, that's how some leaders think, but the journey has just begun.

With every chairperson appointment (especially those who sat in the wrong chairs) comes self-doubt that they can do the job. They lack the confidence and experience, which produces either anxiety or a lack of enthusiasm. Most have no idea how to even run a meeting. What is involved? Who takes the minutes? How do I get everyone to participate? This is the time that a leader needs to switch gears and become a mentor and a coach. Without effective coaching the process is sure to fail. Remember, as a leader, we are only involved in the meetings to support the chair people and to provide the resources to make that committee successful. This is a caregiver lead process. The job of the leader is to make sure the chairperson is successful. Coaching is the key to success. It builds character, instills confidence, and promotes the shared governance model.

I go to every one of the committee meetings, often sitting silent in the back of the room. I don't tell them what to do—I don't give them any tasks but, if asked for my opinion, I will give it. Sometimes I refrain in order to facilitate creative free thinking from the committee.

Reading the Room

Reading the room is a skill that many do not think about when they start their tenure as a chairperson. The ability to "read the room" – to observe the tendencies and behaviors of the meeting participants and to intervene is a skill that needs to be used in a purposeful manner. However, new chair people usually put most of their focus on the task at hand, keeping to the agenda, and making sure they finish on time. Often it is the staff that feel that they are not valued or feel that, based on their job title, they should not speak up. Again, incorporating them into the process helps break down the barriers of role intimidation. This is why reading the room needs to be taught and encouraged.

As meetings proceed, people will start sharing ideas. When they do, the chairperson needs to listen to the idea, while also scanning the room and monitoring others' behaviors. Who's paying attention? Who isn't? Who is involved or not involved?

What do you do with someone who is not paying attention? Maybe they're looking at their phone or talking to the person next to them. I like to deliver my message without words. If a conversation is occurring between two people while I am trying to conduct a meeting, I will stop talking, stand, go over to area where they're sitting, and ask the person sitting next to them to trade seats with me. I don't say anything; I simply sit next to them. This sends the message and quite often, it only takes one seat change for that kind of behavior to never happen again.

Sometimes you have people in the meeting that don't feel like they belong there. They don't think they're "worthy" of being in the room. Those are the people that you need to draw out. Maybe you have a unit clerk or nursing assistant who is sitting there in silence. With this person I might say, "Susan, I know this is something that pertains to you, and I want to hear what you have to say." Then, if they choose to share a thought, encourage them. Ask for more detail. Most of the time the simple acknowledgement will produce an attitude change, and the caregiver will start to be more engaged in the meeting. In addition, you'll see others become more engaged as well.

Reading the room also helps chair people ensure that the meeting stays on track. They need to organize the time to make sure that all of the agenda items are covered during the time allotted. That's not an easy thing to do. It requires the ability to read the room—to control those who over-contribute, draw out those who under-contribute, and to keep the conversation on track. Sometimes conversations will go off track and convert from problem solving to contagious complaining. As the chairperson, you must help the group refocus and stay on task.

Getting Things Done

Not all of the work of a committee gets done during the meetings, of course. Generally what comes out of meetings are tasks that people need to do, information that needs to be gathered, etc. But, what often happens after the meeting?

How long after leaving a meeting you have attended do you think *What do I have to do before the next meeting?* As the chairperson, how do you keep track of what was assigned and who was assigned to it? Many groups rely on meeting minutes. How many people consistently go back and reread meeting minutes to ensure that what they were assigned to do gets done? Not many. What usually happens is the next meeting occurs and someone asks, "Jeff, did you do your assigned task?" Silence from Jeff.

Quite often the idea of what has to be done next gets pushed aside by the tasks of your full time job or what you need to get from the grocery store for dinner. Nothing is more frustrating, and for that matter inefficient, then spending the first 10 minutes of your next committee meeting going over what everyone was supposed to do only to find out half of it was never completed.

In order to help keep chairpeople organized we use the same "Who, What, By When" sheet that we use for the townhalls which was discussed earlier in this book.

The chairperson uses this form to run each meeting. As they move through the meeting, they document who is going to do what, define what "what" is, and by when. At the end of the meeting, they can post this form to remind each person what they are responsible for by the timeframe that was determined by the group.

After the meeting, you take the Who, What, By When sheet, and you post it where it's readily seen. Again, we are excuse busting. A caregiver is no longer able to use the excuse, "I couldn't remember what I was supposed to do for this meeting" When you make a copy and post it where everybody can review or refer to, then the excuse "I forgot what I was supposed to do," is negated.

We have a board that is specifically used for committee information.

Each committee has a portion of the board, and that's where the "Who, What, By When" sheets get posted along with the meeting dates and times for the year as well as any other material that is relevant for that committee, all together in one place. I have had some people tell me they also post the sheets on the intranet and one person told me they attach it to an email and send it to each committee member a week before the next meeting.

In addition to being a reminder, the Who, What by When sheet acts as a meeting organizer. No need to review meeting minutes. When was the last time you attended a meeting and the person running it says, "Let's review last meeting's minutes," and then 6 seconds later, he asks for someone to second the motion to accept them. No one read them! Instead, at the next meeting the chairperson can use the sheet to go down the list of assignments one by one and ask if the person assigned has completed the task. At the same time, you really are reviewing last meeting's minutes. No excuses for those who did not complete their tasks. If someone fails to do what he or she was assigned, they're called out in the meeting. It is peer accountability rather than leadership mandates.

You Snooze, You Lose

Getting people to volunteer for assignments just means that you are giving them more work. Although this cannot be argued, the reality is that it is work that is required to make the real work that they do even easier. So, it is in their best interest to participate. But this is still not enough of an incentive for some to volunteer. This is often a great frustration for chair people. When coaching them, I advise them to use the "you snooze, you lose" approach.

What I encourage chair people to do is list the "fun" agenda items which need action taken, first. Why? Because the people who are your best meeting participants, the ones who are engaged and energetic, are likely to volunteer first for assignments or sub groups. They should be rewarded for their eager participation. When you get to the less fun things, for example, "who wants to review policies for accuracy?" you can assign that to someone who hasn't volunteered yet. "Hey, Bob. I haven't really heard from you much. Since you're the only committee member who hasn't volunteered yet, I will ask that you help with this task." This encourages all participants to volunteer early and be an active participant in the meeting. Sometimes, I will assign tasks that no one in attendance wants to do or assign it to a person who never attends the meetings. That's right, I'll call them on the phone and say, "Sorry to see you didn't get to the meeting today. We needed someone to do chart audits, and you were assigned to help complete this." People quickly figure out that it is in their best interest to be active or they'll be assigned a task that no one else wants to do.

Everyone participates. Everyone has a say. If you don't speak up, then you forego your right to tell us how you think the current program isn't working. You have to earn that right. We're talking about participating in 50 percent of the meetings, which only last an hour, and are only once a month. That's only *6 hours* a year. If you can't commit to that minimal amount of time, then it's time to find another hospital.

Once the caregivers are on board and they attend their first meeting, they see the dynamics and the culture that we have in place. They see that these committees do exist and are empowered to make real change. Caregivers are held accountable to the process and when they see that this isn't just smoke and mirrors, they become engaged in the process. This is real caregiver engagement.

Meeting After the Meeting

After the first meeting of a committee, I will meet privately with the leadership group. I'll call together the manager, the clinical liaison, and the chairperson, and I'll say, "How do you think that meeting went?" I'll listen to their perspectives, often prompting them for more information. If they say, "It went well," I'll probe for more detail. I'll ask, "What one particular thing popped into your head just now when you said that?" I'll keep probing until I get some specifics. I'll share my perspectives, "You're right. I think it did go well. For a first meeting, I thought it was great."

I'll follow up on this by asking, "What could have been done better?" I want to see if the chairperson has any personal insight as to how the meeting truly went. What was the overall feeling? What were some of your favorite ideas presented today? Who wasn't involved? How did you involve the people on the phone? These are all questions that stimulate a different kind of thinking. These are group leader thoughts which differ from meeting participant thoughts.

If the feeling was that not everyone participated, I'll then ask: What could you have done to get them involved? Did you remember to assign tasks to those not in attendance? These are important to address.

Remember that we want to recognize and reward those individuals who actively participate in meetings. We often assign important tasks to the hard workers who are on our team. Why? Because we know the task will get done and it will get done the right way. But what are we really doing? We are giving more and more work to the optimistic positive caregiver while we are essentially excluding and excusing the slackers from work that needs to get done. There needs to be a balance here. Avoid this common pitfall and spread the tasks out evenly.

Remember, help the chair people to succeed and allow the caregivers to make decisions that directly affect their working environment. This is empowerment and with empowerment comes engagement.

FINALLY, CULTURE CHANGE!

So, how do you know when your culture has finally changed for the better? How do you know when you have motivation and empowerment? There are a number of signs that it has happened.

You know you have achieved that balance of motivation and empowerment when staff see themselves as being accountable to the unit and their fellow colleagues. It happens when the caregivers seek out opportunities to shine without limitation and when conflicts are resolved among people without blame. You have true engagement when the caregivers independently find issues that need to be addressed, and then work together to find solutions to those problems. I love watching it. It's what fuels me as a leader.

I like to refer to these observations as "tie moments." They're moments when I feel so proud of the group. For being independent. For having pride in what they do and accepting accountability for its results. It brings a tear to my eye, and I need to lift my necktie to my face to blot my tears. It's what leadership is all about.

CHAPTER 6
BELIEVE, BELIEVE, BELIEVE

It is important to continuously remind yourself that your culture did not sour overnight. Your attempt to change the culture will not be painless and it will take time. Not every caregiver is going to be successful. Not every caregiver who signed the Clinical Excellence Commitment Board is going to uphold that commitment. Not every caregiver assigned to a committee is going to be a high-performing team member.

The first step in achieving true caregiver engagement is to understand the journey. Leadership is an attitude and it takes guts and determination to pursue this journey. This mindset will help you to push through the inevitable difficult times and to develop a contagious positive attitude that others will want to follow. Believe, believe, believe not only in yourself, but in the positive caregivers that want the same as you and a successful healthcare team that nurtures and supports each other for the benefit of the patients and their families.

As a leader, your role is to be clear about expectations, to get commitments from your employees to meet those expectations, to provide coaching and counseling to help them be successful, and to hold them accountable and take steps to course correct. If career relocation for the caregiver becomes necessary, then you can take some solace in the fact that you believed in them until you just couldn't anymore.

GIVE THEM EVERY OPPORTUNITY TO SUCCEED

If you want people to work for you, then you have to work for them. A philosophy of "giving the caregivers the opportunity to succeed" is important here. You have to believe in them, every one of them, even the low performers. Why? Because they deserve it. If you keep that philosophy then—not only will you watch some of the low performers step up and amaze you—you will also be a much happier and optimistic leader.

As you begin to assess the abilities of your caregiver team, you will discover that not all caregivers are the same. In his book, *Good to Great*, Jim Collins uses a bus analogy to identify three categories of employees that leaders generally find themselves working with.

- *High performers.* These are the caregivers that sit in the front of the bus driving it to greatness. They are the ones who lead everyone else. They feel a personal responsibility to ensure success and to lead the department in the right direction. They are those that look to exceed expectations, not just simply meet them. This is the group that needs to be celebrated and fostered. They are the favorites that the underperformers fear because they set the bar of success too high for them to reach. Often the other groups consider them the "favorites" when in reality they are the ones who should be celebrated for always going above and beyond expectations.

- *Middle performers.* These are the caregivers who sit in the middle of the bus. They come in, do their jobs, and go home. Unlike the apathetic 20 percenters discussed later in the chapter, this group is usually hardworking and loyal to the team. They take pride in the job that they do but offer nothing more. You appreciate them because they are the quiet caregivers who just get it done. They consistently meet expectations, but consider it an effort to exceed them. My experience is that some will rise to the occasion if given the opportunity whereas others will run when asked to volunteer.

- *Low performers.* These are the caregivers that sit in the back of the bus. They are given every opportunity to succeed, hoping to at least move them to the middle of the bus. They are the 20 percenters, a group of caregivers who purposefully underperform and eagerly attempt to destroy the culture that you are trying to build. They are the ones that sit in the breakroom and talk about ways to defeat every program you come up with, or worse, defeat you as a leader. Leaders often make the mistake of spending most of their time trying to discipline and change the behavior of this group. This doesn't mean we need to give up on the low performers. Again, believe, believe, believe and always give the caregivers every chance to succeed.[23]

Have Faith

I like to approach leadership from the perspective of believing in people and taking an optimistic, rather than a pessimistic, view of what they're capable of doing. It takes a lot less energy to do things that way than to spend your time worrying about their negative behavior. If you focus your energy on the positive individuals, then that spirit and enthusiasm eventually prevails. The reason why that is not the case is because many leaders focus most of their energy on the negative caregivers, or what I call the 20 percenters. They never shift their focus to the 80 percent (the positive caregivers). We only focus on the 20 percenters (the negative caregivers) and then optimism and enthusiasm for the positive dies because no leader is there to encourage and nurture it.

Trust me, the 20 percenters will persist and even try to convert others to their pessimistic ways. There is a portion of this group who will either be inspired by the energy of the 80 percent or see that being negative will not be tolerated anymore, and it will change their ways. It takes more energy to be happy then it does to be negative, but the positive energy is so much stronger. If in the end you can't convert them, you will at least know that you gave them every chance to be successful. You are not a failure if this doesn't occur, but you are a disappointment if you allow the negativity to persist. Give them every chance to succeed, they may surprise you!

There are always ways for leaders to help motivate the 20 percenters, many of which are found throughout this book. Identifying whether or not they have the ability to be better is a good first step. If they lack the basic skills or desire to exceed their current effort, then the likelihood of future success is small. I believe that sometimes you need to give lower performers more responsibility. I know it is counterintuitive, but we do this for two reasons. The first is that sometimes people avoid responsibility because they lack the confidence needed to perform well. Sometimes providing menial tasks to be completed by the individual and then acknowledging and

---

[23] Collins, J. (2001). *Good to Great: Why some companies make the leap…and others don't.* New York, NY: Harper Collins.

thanking them for completing the task can motivate low performers to want to do more.

A good example of this is when I was a new nurse. I wasn't a very good nurse. As a matter of fact, I would call myself a lazy low performer, part of the 20 percent crowd. My former manager gave me a menial task to complete despite the fact that I showed little effort to perform the basic tasks assigned to me on a daily basis. She simply asked me to relabel all of the drawers in each room so that each room looked the same. A simple task, that once completed and acknowledged, inspired me to do more. I believe it is what sparked the leadership bug within myself a long time ago.

Another positive outcome to giving the low performers more work to do is the boost it gives the high performers when they see that the work is being shared and that they are not the only ones being asked to perform duties above and beyond what is considered their day-to-day tasks. Think about who is the most overworked person on your unit? It is the caregiver who always does a great job when assigned a task? Is that person usually a high performer? These high performing caregivers are often taxed with added responsibilities because leaders know they will do the job and do it right. Meanwhile, the 20 percenters that do a bad job are never asked to do anything extra. It's like being married and asked to do a load of whites. Some men (not me, of course!) throw a red item of clothing in there, turn the whole load pink, and suddenly, no more laundry for him! Give the low performers continuous opportunities to step up. They will either live up to the culture of the department or they will be exposed and eventually asked to move on.

The 20 Percenters

This is a book about positivity, empowerment, and staff engagement. Keeping to this vision, I have tried to maintain the focus on the 80 percent of the caregivers who want to be a part of the culture change. As much as I would like to keep the focus on them, the reality is that there are individuals within every department who do not agree with department philosophies or who are unwilling to change. There are a few in this group that will eventually see that the positivity will win out and so they join the 80 percent; however, there are a few that will not. So, I will take just a small portion of this book to help leaders identify who the 20 percenters are and how to handle them. Of course, the best option is to always try to believe, believe, believe and help them become at least middle performers, but, when that fails, something else needs to be done.

Who are the 20 percenters? You probably have a picture of someone's face in your brain as you read this paragraph. There are those that hide in the shadows, causing mischief in little secret huddles that suddenly stop as you walk by while there are some that don't hide at all. Both groups try to recruit others into their circle of negativity. As a leader, it's important for you to identify them, if not for yourself, do it on behalf of the positive caregivers that are held hostage by their behavior. Table 6.1 identifies and categorizes some key behaviors of the 20 percenters.

Table 6.1 Negativity in the Workplace: The Twenty Percent			
Negative Behavior Identification	What they do	Why they do it	How to fix it
Resistance	• Traditionalists who prefer the status quo • Masters of delay who stall the process of change • Do anything they can to resist the change • Do not usually recruit others	• May feel forced to change their practice too often without any input in the process • May have tenure and a sense of entitlement • May feel a need for change means the way they previously worked is somehow wrong	• Meet with and acknowledge their concerns • Help them to understand how the changes may benefit them • Encourage active participation on committees to control the change • Education, communication, and if that fails remediation
Apathy	• Attend work to complete their job and head home without a sense of engagement • Drag everyone down because they do not partake in the synergistic group working toward	• Often they are senior nurses close to retirement • May include younger nurses who are used to instant gratification and settle into status quo when it does	• Assign easily accomplished tasks to ensure success • Identify a strength in these individuals and capitalize on it, i.e., precepting • Mentor these individuals to

Table 6.1 Negativity in the Workplace: The Twenty Percent			
Negative Behavior Identification	What they do	Why they do it	How to fix it
	excellence • They strive to meet a goal, not to exceed it • Often strong clinically and use that as their badge of honor	not occur • Purposeful noncompliance to prove their dissatisfaction	determine if another area of work or location within the hospital would better suit their personality
Cynicism	• Question everything without offering any solutions • First to say, "That's never going to work!" • Deflate any excitement a change might generate	• Previous experience with leaders who did not follow through • Committed to programs in the past that failed	• A serious effort to repair trust • Chipping away at the low-hanging fruit, which are the small things a leader can immediately address as a sign of good faith
Spite	• Examine loopholes in current policies with the intention to exploit them • Manipulate situations by using anything said or written verbatim to make a point • Usually feel angry and bitter	• Previous success undermining other leaders • This negative behavior attracts others, which strengthens the impact of the negative behaviors • Like to always be right	• Be well versed in the policies and always present facts • Don't fight and give energy to the loophole, just close it • Education, communication, and, if that fails, remediation
Sabotage	• Intent is to undermine leadership efforts • Create roadblocks to halt or call into	• Pure anger at a leader, policy or a change • A sense of power when	• Rely on the 80 percent to inform you of the individuals who are responsible

Table 6.1 Negativity in the Workplace: The Twenty Percent			
Negative Behavior Identification	What they do	Why they do it	How to fix it
	question any new idea • Recruit others to assist them	successful • Negative energy gives them power	• Empower the positive caregivers to be champions for the change • Be aware of side meetings or conversations that suddenly stop when you are in the vicinity

Be Prepared With the Facts

There are many times when caregivers may come to you with an issue, or you may be informed that they want to talk with you about a concern. When this happens, I like to be prepared. I like to do some background research and gather some facts before the meeting. It is always good to ask your leadership team if they have heard anything about the issue that the caregiver is about to talk with you about. If so, this may give you an opportunity to research the issue and be prepared with the facts needed to form a communication strategy. The strategy is to understand the true issue, identify challenges that the caregiver is about to present, and perhaps have an answer or a solution to the problem. Knowing the facts gives you the knowledge you need to counter argue the point or perhaps defuse the situation.

For example, I worked with Alex, a volunteer paramedic who would regularly work his paramedic job at night and then come work for us in the Emergency Department during the day. He was late all the time. *All* the time! And, although I respect the job that he did volunteering as a paramedic, he was constantly letting his fellow caregivers down. So, I called him into my office and I said, "Alex, you've been late for the twelfth time. This is your final written warning." He paused and replied, "Charles, I just want to call your attention to Pennsylvania Statute #52967—that states that any volunteer paramedic, if engaged in performing his duties as a volunteer paramedic, cannot be penalized for fulfilling his responsibilities."

Unprepared and without the facts, I was forced to take him at his word.

He had me. Or did he? Anticipating another lateness to occur in the near future, I prepared myself with the facts. Alex was indeed late again for the 13th time just 3 weeks later. I called him into my office, and he immediately reminded me of Statute #52967. The only problem for Alex was that I was now prepared with the facts. I had pulled the statute prior to our meeting. I pointed out to Alex that he'd left out an important part of the statute during our earlier discussion—the part that says that if you're late, you need to provide a note from the Squad Chief stating that he had indeed had a late call on the day in question. I then informed Alex he had until Monday to produce 13 notes.

I talk about giving everyone a chance and believing in people. I wanted to believe that all of the tardiness was truly caused by Alex doing his duties at the ambulance squad. This is why Alex got 12 additional opportunities. It is unfortunate though that some individuals will take advantage of liberties and test your knowledge as a leader. Being prepared with the facts will help you to keep you focus on the real issue, what is good for all of the caregivers, not just one.

After asking for the notes required by law it was apparent that Alex wasn't prepared. It was clear that Alex was manipulating the situation to his advantage and stretching the truth and hoping that I did not come to our meetings prepared with the facts. So, you need to take the time to gather information so you're prepared. Yes, this may take some additional work up front, but, in the long run, it will be well worth the effort.

Alex didn't have a note. He couldn't produce 13 of them by Monday. He had gotten numerous chances to succeed. Alex was working the system and using a loophole. We tried to help motivate Alex to become a high performer. We gave him opportunities to exceed expectations. Despite our best efforts, Alex continued to try to manipulate the system. It is unfortunate, but it is a reality. There will be some that you cannot motivate or empower to be a part of the culture you are trying to establish. Alex doesn't work for us any longer.

Be Okay With Silence

They say silence is golden; I say it is a very effective leadership communication tool. As leaders, we need to learn to be comfortable with silence, but it can be tough to do. Leaders often feel an obligation to fill those uncomfortable silent gaps with caregivers. So, as compassionate individuals, we will empathize with someone when a crucial conversation is occurring, and we'll fill in the blanks for them when silence occurs; we'll jump in to finish their sentences. This is basically giving them a get-out-of-jail-free card instead of using the opportunity to utilize a very powerful leadership skill, silence. For instance, often times I will call a caregiver into my office and ask them why they think I called them into the office. After I ask the question, I remain silent and make eye contact. It is typical that they remain silent as well. The reality is that inside their heads, they are the opposite of silent. They are doing a rapid fire question session. They may be asking themselves:

> Did I do something wrong that I don't know about?
> Does he know about the ACE bandage I took home for my mom?
> Does he know I was really at the beach when I called in last week?
> If he does know and I admit it, will I get leniency?
> If I admit to it and that's not what he is talking about, then I will give myself away for no reason.

The questions are endless and with each moment of their silence, the questions become more intense.

Silence is a particularly effective tool to handle rumor control. For example, you hear that Kathy has been taking supplies from the closet for her own personal use. You confirm this by completing inventory and see that only orthopedic supplies are missing. A number of people have reported Kathy is taking the supplies, but they don't have proof. An effective way to handle this type of situation is to call Kathy into the office and simply state, "You know why I called you in here today." Then, let the silence begin. After a good pause, I will often ask a follow up question such as, "Anything I should know or that you want to tell me?" More silence. Learn to become comfortable with silence. Give people time to think. Use it as a tool to deliver messages. Even if Kathy does not admit to stealing the supplies, you as a leader, have indirectly communicated the message that you are aware of these events and now you're watching. In most instances, the behavior will stop.

Make Sure the Punishment Fits the Crime

Everything should be relative to the action performed. You're not going to give a written warning to someone you find texting at the nurse's station for the first time. On the other hand, you're also not going to give a verbal warning to a nurse that takes a swing at a nursing assistant. The punishment must fit the crime. If the punishment is too strict, the leader may be seen as vindictive. Caregivers may be afraid to take any risks in fear of serious consequences. You don't want to prevent caregivers from taking initiative like the emergency room technician did when she completed another EKG on a patient she felt needed it, even though the circumstances prevented seeking timely permission. If she feared that there would be extreme consequences for taking that risk, she would have been less likely to break the rules. Although accountability is needed, serious punishment that doesn't fit the infraction deters caregivers from taking risks that bring value to the patient experience. On the other hand, if the consequence is too lenient, the deterring effect of the punishment will be diminished.

Consistency comes into play here, again, as do your Commitment Standards. What are the expectations? What are the consequences? Communicate them. Follow them consistently!

Have a Short Memory

When you're in a leadership role, you need to have a short memory. Focus on the issue that is presented to you and give the caregiver opportunities for improvement. Once the conversation is over, move on. Don't hang on, and certainly don't let that conversation affect any future conversation you may have with that same caregiver. Each issue is independent unless the behavior becomes a pattern.

This is also important for the mental health of the leader. If you can't let the issues go, burnout will occur. Realize people make mistakes. Continue to support and believe in each caregiver.

WHEN ALL ELSE FAILS

Let's face it. Despite all of your best efforts, there may be some people who you cannot convert to the positive culture you are trying to build. If this is the case, then it may be time to career relocate them. This can be very stressful for leaders, but there are things that leaders can do to be prepared to have the difficult conversation. New leaders often mention they have anxiety and outright fear when it is time to fire someone. To help leaders deal with the anxiety, I offer them the following thoughts.

> ➤ If you have completed your job as a leader and provided your colleague every opportunity to succeed, then you can have

confidence in your decision.

> During your last meeting with your colleague, did you inform them of the consequences that could lead to firing should that behavior happen again?

> Did you provide every resource possible (for example, an employee assistance program or encouragement to join a self-governance committee) to help them be successful?

Help Them Move On

If you have completed everything discussed in this chapter, then the termination meeting should be relatively easy even if you dread it. If at every step of the disciplinary process you said, "Tom, I just want to let you know, you have two more chances." Then the next time, "Tom you need to know that the next time this occurs, you will receive a final written warning." And, finally, "Tom, the next time this occurs we will be parting ways. Do you understand that?" If you have been very clear with expectations, then the final meeting should be relatively brief. Tom already knows why you are asking him to come to the office.

In these situations, when I ask the caregiver if they know why I brought them in, they will inevitably say, "Yes, I guess I'm fired." I will respond, "Yes, that's right. Unfortunately, we talked about this, and we discussed that the next time this occurred, I would have no choice. I have done everything I could for you. I've made every attempt to be able to support you and provide you with the resources you need, but this hasn't worked so, yes, we're terminating your employment with us today." Most of the time, they don't argue. They just turn in their ID, and they walk out the door.

If you're not finding this to be the case, then you need to look at your own leadership practices to determine why they don't understand. What messages have you failed to deliver?

CHAPTER 7
CREATIVELY CELEBRATING SUCCESS

Having celebrations and recognizing staff has always been an important part of leadership. I remember going through training where I was taught that sending a handwritten thank you letter to a caregiver was a gesture that could make a positive difference. As mentioned in Chapter 2, there are some that are thankful for this type of appreciative act, but there are some that will feel it is not enough. Finding what motivates each individual is important. Of course, caregivers love to be recognized, but if there is no creativity in the methods you use, then the meaning starts to fade and so does the positive affect it has in building team morale.

So, what can a leader do to avoid this decline? First, you can get over the feeling that "The staff is ungrateful because they didn't like your thank-you note," or that "They're upset that it's just another t-shirt." I would be overly optimistic if I thought there would be a time when everyone was always thankful. Regardless of the few negative individuals, a leader must do what they think is right, simply because it is the right thing to do. Don't let the naysayers discourage you from celebrating successes. The positive caregivers (80 percenters) deserve to be acknowledged, so consider it a leadership opportunity to do the right thing.

Remember that rewards and recognition send a signal to the caregivers that you value who they are and what they are doing. Positive acknowledgement reinforces positive behavior, which makes it more likely that the behavior will be repeated in the future. It is the fuel of culture change, and without it the quest for real culture change will fail. Motivation comes in many forms and understanding what motivates each individual can benefit a leader.

IN THE MOMENT RECOGNITION

Whether it is a pizza party to celebrate reaching your patient satisfaction goal or a simple "thank you" card after a very busy shift, the In the Moment Recognition (IMR) reward provides an immediate acknowledgement of a job well done. This extrinsic form of motivation should not be relied on as the only form of motivation. As discussed in Chapter 2, extrinsic motivation can be limited in its effectiveness over an extended period of time so it must be used wisely. When caregivers receive material rewards, such as pizza, there is an immediate material value, and, if not overdone, an emotional value or intrinsic response can be realized. Creativity helps to energize these types of reward and recognition programs and helps a leader find different ways to immediately recognize the team. It doesn't have to be an expensive endeavor; it simply has to acknowledge a job well done.

CREATIVELY FOSTERING SUCCESS

Any reward program can be successful if you tap into the creativity and imagination of the caregivers. Finding fun ways to celebrate daily achievements with a simple gesture is a great way to foster team building while achieving the goals set for the department. For example, the Colleague Engagement Committee wanted to celebrate those who always smiled. The feeling was that a smile can be contagious, so why not put one on your face? (The committee thought that was a fun slogan.) So, we assigned certain undercover smile agents who would put a little sticker on your ID if they thought you were a good smiler that shift. Creative and inexpensive, this program produced positive recognition while increasing our smile quota.

These are the types of programs that help to sustain a team's momentum while they pursue culture change. Earlier in this book, we discussed a leader's need to understand that with change comes anxiety and the possibility of regression before real culture change is realized. Just the fact that a leader is encouraging the free-thinking to brainstorm support programs is seen as an attempt to support caregivers through this difficult process. The following programs are some of the most creative and inspiring programs that I have had the pleasure of being a part of as a leader. They are caregiver-inspired, sustainable, and inexpensive to implement.

Beads for Deeds Program

The first program ever to be developed by our colleague engagement committee was called the Beads for Deeds program. Its origin began when the committee was challenged to find a way to improve caregiver satisfaction and morale across all disciplines. I assigned them this goal because, in my short tenure as the manager of the emergency department, I had made an observation about the social structure of the caregivers. It was apparent that each discipline that worked in the ER worked within their own silo, meaning they only socialized with people who were like them. The nurses hung out with and supported the other nurses. The techs did the same, feeling they needed to support and protect each other. The physicians barely communicated to anyone, including the nurses. Everyone lived and practiced within their silos.

There was a distinct hierarchy of abuse. Doctors talked down to the nurses. Nurses disrespected the ED techs. The techs needed to find a way to be heard so they spoke poorly to the unit clerks. Yes, the poor unit clerks had no one to pick on.

We needed a way to break those walls down, but how do you change a culture that's been in place for 20 years? The Colleague Engagement Committee (formally called the fun committee) thought a good way to do this was to create a program that promoted peer recognition among colleagues. The committee referred to the program as a silo buster. The idea was to provide the opportunity to recognize good deeds that exceed expectations across all disciplines. Another goal for this program was to make it peer-to-peer recognition as opposed to leadership driven. They also wanted the acknowledgement to be public. When examining other employee recognition programs, they noticed that recognition was often given to caregivers without public celebration and the board that acknowledged these accomplishments was often found in the staff lounge where no one other than the caregivers could see it.

Beads for Deeds works as follows. First, anytime someone identifies another caregiver who has gone above and beyond expectations, they nominate them by filling out a Beads for Deeds slip. That slip goes into a box and a multidisciplinary subcommittee of three take the ballots and determine bead worthiness. Most beads are awarded, but there are, at times, one or two that don't quite live up to the spirit of the program are disqualified. For example, the committee once received the following nomination.

"I am nominating Sue because she remembered that I love Mochaccino Mondays, and she got me one."

Although this was very nice of Sue, it was not an exceptional gesture. Another example of a rejected bead included this submission, *"Jamie agreed to stay late for me when I was running late for my shift."* Although this was nice of Jamie, the deed does not go above and beyond the expectation.

Going above and beyond is the key here. For example, the following bead was rewarded for going beyond what was expected. During the week of Christmas, an ER tech named Sally made "Reindeer food," consisting of oats and glitter, to give to sick kids visiting the Emergency Department. She would use the story of how magical this reindeer food was in order to distract sick and frightened children during procedures.

Once the committee approves the bead, the person nominated receives one blue bead. This bead is placed on a wine ring (the kind you use to identify your glass of wine at a party), and then it is secured to your badge. Once you get to five blue beads (five good deeds), then you have a choice. You can trade in those five blue beads for a prize or trade them in for a green bead, which has a higher value with better prizes. The prize for trading in blue beads is nominal. Sort of like when you go to the arcade and win tickets. 100 tickets gets you a plastic spider, while 1000 tickets gets you a pencil and some Twizzlers. The catch is that if you trade in your beads for a prize, then you start again with zero beads.

Once you 5 five green beads you can trade them in for 1 red or select a prize with greater value. Same rules apply. If you get 5 red beads, you can trade it in for the coveted pearl bead (that's 125 good deeds). The prize for the pearl is a half a day off (got your attention now?), but that can only happen if you trade them in.

The program started, and, just as I expected, the docs nominated docs, the nurses nominated nurses, right down the line. The committee's intention to break down the silos was not working. This went on for about a month and then something wonderful happened. A doctor, who at times could be a bit gruff, nominated a tech for something they had done. It was the talk of the town. "Did you hear what happened? The doctor nominated Dawn!" The others could not believe it. "She did? Really, she nominated a tech?" It was the one small gesture needed to start breaking down those walls. Before we knew it, RNs were nominating unit clerks, and techs were nominating docs. The walls were starting to crumble, and it was wonderful to watch.

Communication started to improve among the caregivers. Instead of orders, there were requests. Clinical demands were replaced with collegial support. Mutual respect was starting to develop, and, instead of working in silos, caregivers were now working together as a team. They shared one common goal, which was providing compassionate care to all patients and their families. This type of engagement removed the barriers and created an environment where people wanted to work together.

When I travel the country for various speaking engagements, I like to ask organizations if they have staff recognition programs. They often answer "yes" quickly and with pride. I ask them to show it to me, and without fail, they walk me into the staff lounge. There are some beautiful acknowledgement boards. I always follow up, "Who gets to see this board?" They answer, "The staff does." Success in this type of program cannot be solely measured by the satisfaction of the caregiver. True success translates to the experience of the patient. Let me explain.

Because the beads in our program are on a ring, which is placed around your ID, it is right out there in the open for patients and their families to see. Patients get to ask, "What are those beads?" Caregivers have the opportunity to tell the patient all the great things that they have done that helped them get the beads. This not only instills confidence in the patient that their caregiver has been recognized for the great things they have done, but it also instills a sense of pride in the colleague who gets to tell the patient and their families about all of their recognized accomplishments. It's a win-win.

Let me give you another example of how this type of recognition instills confidence in others. Imagine that you are going into battle. You look to your right and see a private like yourself, proud and strong but not a lot of medals to prove his experience. You look to your left and you see a highly decorated soldier with medals that show his bravery and competence. Which of these two would you feel comfortable following into battle? Now, I know fighting in a war and working in healthcare cannot be seriously compared, but the effect is similar in that recognition programs which publicly acknowledge caregivers can instill confidence in those around them.

On average, about 5 beads are awarded every 2 weeks. Obviously, this can vary. After review, very few are rejected now that there is an understanding of what constitutes a bead. The committee has a rule that if there is any question as to whether a nomination is bead-worthy, then the bead is to be given. It has to be unanimous that it is not a valid nomination for it to be rejected. To become picky and reject the nomination would create a negative feeling about a positive program.

For those thinking *I can't afford to do that program*, let me lay out the costs for you. This program costs $26 for the supplies (rings and beads) and $500 for the prizes. That's it. The natural question is, what happens if people keep handing in their beads for prizes? That $500 worth of prizes will dissipate quickly and the program will cost more over time. In my experience the opposite happens. Our program has been in place since 2003 and only one person has traded in their beads for a prize. Only *one*. Apparently pride and collegial competition was more important than movie passes. Love it!

T.O.P. (Team Oriented People) Teams

Now that the silos are starting to fall, the team was tasked with another challenge. How do we continue to strengthen our ability to work together as a team? This challenge is straightforward. Leadership's only parameter assigned to the caregivers was the idea that whatever program they came up with needed to be fun as well as effective.

In order to get started, we needed to understand what success looks like. So the committee developed a program we referred to as the T.O.P. (Team Oriented People) Teams. These teams were challenged to work together as a team to keep the department JCAHO-ready at all times. You know what JCAHO-ready means, right? It's the scramble that occurs when the Joint Commission or Department of Health shows up at the front door for a surprise visit. The department never looks as good as it does then. Don't you wish the department looked that good all the time? Well, there are fun ways to make that happen while also building teamwork and collaboration.

This is how the T.O.P. program works. At the time, I had five others on my leadership team. I informed them that each leader was about to get a chance to lead a group of people and do great things. I explained that their team would be assigned to a geographical location of the department. Each team would be responsible to keep that area JCAHO-ready at all times. That means keeping it clean, putting in work orders to fix broken furniture, ordering supplies, and keeping their area stocked. Each of these teams were responsible for their section of the department. This program afforded me the opportunity to coach my young leaders while the success of each team provided a sense of pride for a job well done.

In a private location the program began by handing out 5 lists to each leader. The first list was a list of the unit clerks who worked in our department. We drew numbers out of hat to see which leader would pick first. The first leader picked the unit clerk they felt would be best on their team from the list, and the other leaders followed until all of the unit clerks were picked. We did this for each discipline, and, in the end, each leader had a team made up of unit clerks, techs, nurses, physician assistants, and, yes, *even* doctors. The rules were simple. Keep your area JCAHO-ready. To add a little fun to the program each team was asked to name their teams whatever they wanted, and if they needed resources, they needed to ask. I would hold each leader accountable, and that leader was responsible to hold each of their team members to the same expectation. It was the leader's responsibility to educate, coach, and hold accountable their team. The hope was that coaching the leaders would help them to coach their own team members. This is also a great way to develop future leaders and lends itself to developing a successful succession plan.

Some of the teams got creative and had fun with it. Some of the names of the teams were entertaining. The team assigned to the trauma area named their team "the Trauma Junkies." One team named themselves the "Scrubbing Bubbles." We even had one team that called themselves "M&Ms with no nuts." Not sure what that meant or how they came up with that one, but creativity is always welcomed, just as long as it's fun and respectful.

Each month, a panel of judges inspected and ranked the five areas for cleanliness, organization, and efficiency. Sometimes I would be the sole judge. To make it fun, I would wear a sash or a top hat while judging. Of course, discretion is required so that patients don't misconstrue the meaning of the judging. Other times, I would enlist guest judges such as the CNO or better yet the plumber from plant operations. Sometimes, there were secret shopper judges on off shifts. We asked volunteers and one time we even asked a family member, who had inquired what the guy in the sash (me) was doing, to be a judge once.

Initially, after judging, we picked a first place winner and an underachiever. The first place winners were rewarded with one assignment switch card each. This card allowed them to switch their assignment any time over the course of the next month. You can imagine how valuable the switch cards were to the teams. The underachievers had to work in triage or sub-acute, the two least favorable assignments for a week.

Some lessons are learned through errors. Just as we picked the winner we also identified the loser. Isolating an underachieving team was meant to motivate, but, unfortunately, it did the opposite. It discouraged the enthusiasm of the program and some people quit trying, including upset winners who felt it was not right to make a loser out of people who were trying. I quickly changed the last rule. I learned a very valuable lesson that day:

Never put a negative consequence into a positive program.

The TOP Teams were designed to encourage teamwork and promote effective processes to keep our unit inspection ready. We needed a way to test whether we could make that happen, but we needed to do it without making the staff feel like they were being tested. The answer to making that a possibility, of course, was to make it fun.

The game we created was called code PARCO (which is backward for what you would normally say when the Department of Health shows up unexpectedly). The education committee created a system and trained the caregivers. If a surprise inspection should occur the charge RN would go to the drawer, grab the folder and then hand out preassigned task sheets to individuals on each team. These tasks are listed in priority order and once completed that caregiver is to report back to the charge nurse that their duties are complete. If they cannot complete a task, the caregiver must report that immediately to the person in charge so that a different plan can be made. Divide and conquer!

In order to ensure that we had this process perfected I would randomly test the system. I would call a PARCO during the day and hide in a room and watch the magic happen. I would set my alarm for 2am and call in a PARCO. Sometimes, I would go back to sleep, and sometimes I would actually go in. I would call it on the weekends as well as the occasional holiday. The point here is, we had fun with it.

The rewards of this program were two-fold. First, the department was always close, if not actually, ready for a surprise inspection. There was a pride among the teams knowing that their area was prepared and that they worked together to achieve this result. I will tell you that if I called a PARCO today on any of my departments, they could be inspection-ready within 20 minutes. A second unforeseen benefit of this program occurred, when we noticed that our patient satisfaction scores were improving. Patients and their families noted the cleanliness and organization of the department. This indeed improved the patient experience. This was only possible because the staff were engaged in the process. They were competing against each other and at the same time, creating an environment for patients to heal. It demonstrated the true connection between caregiver engagement and transforming the patient experience.

Golden Urinal Awards

What's a golden urinal, you ask? It's one of our most creative and fun programs created to help to celebrate all of our caregivers. It is an inexpensive way to break down silos and celebrate success, and the staff love it. This festive award ceremony occurs during Emergency Nurses Week. However, we don't call it Nurses Week, because that would alienate the other caregivers that work in the department. We simply call it ER week. It's a week to celebrate our team of healthcare professionals, all of them.

The awards ceremony preparation actually occurs two months prior to the actual ceremony. At that time the leadership team comes together to create award categories that are then posted for all caregivers to write in their vote. The categories have three main themes:

Humorous
"Charge nurse with the darkest blackest cloud that follows her"
"ER tech most likely to get pooped on"
"Queen or King of the Rectal temp" (Given to the physician that loves to order a rectal temp despite the age or complaint of the patient).

Inspiring
"Physician you want to see standing above you if your life was in peril"
"Nurse who is the go-to person for any question"

"Unit Clerk who is the best multitasker"
"Tech you want standing next to you when a patient is crashing"

And the "best of"
Nurse of the year (This person gets to attend the ENA national conference)
Tech of the year
Unit clerk of the year
Physician Assistant of the year
Doc of the year

We try to change the categories each year to keep it fresh. After the write-in ballots are complete, they are handed in to the nurse manager. The results are tabulated and the top three finalists from each category are announced and listed under each question, and the new ballots are sent back to the caregivers. The caregivers choose from the three finalists in each category and they are sent back to the manager where she records the winner. We do this two-step process because we learned early on that if people believed they had a chance to win, they were more likely to attend the awards ceremony.

We prepare for the awards banquet by reallocating a few urinals from the supply closet. Little tip: If you take two urinals from the supply closet every month, administration will never know they are missing! Or you could repurpose used ones, but that's kind of gross! We then spray paint them gold. A team of caregivers called the crafters take the urinals and decorate them in ways that celebrate each category. Each award has its own themed urinal.

Some other things that we do to prepare for the awards are as follows: The staff collects pictures, which were captured throughout the year, and we create a slide show set to music. We also work with our local nursing home community to make centerpieces for the tables, as well as chip in to buy prizes for a gift basket, which is raffled off during the banquet.

In the old days, we would partner with a drug company to supply the meal, but that is no longer allowed. No problem. We found a fun way to fix that issue, with a competition, of course! Each member of the leadership team, nursing and physicians, pick a meal course out a hat. There are 9 of us, so 3 will pick "make an appetizer", 3 others will choose "a main course", and the last 3 have "make a dessert". As each caregiver enters the ceremony, they are given three individual pieces of candy corn. They get to sample each of the food choices, and then they drop a single candy corn into the cup that sits in front of their favorite appetizer, main course, and dessert. The leader with the most candy corn in their category wins and has bragging rights for a year.

During the actual ceremony, I don a top hat and grab the microphone. During the event, we tell jokes and funny stories from the year. We give out the urinals and the recipients feel appreciated. I am always amazed at how serious people take the event. They won't share who they voted for and the nominees show up in force.

Pretty fun idea, right? It's fun, but more importantly, this event is another way to break down our silos and celebrate each other. You can write as many thank-you cards as you want, but if you want people to appreciate each other, it needs to go beyond the administration suite. This peer recognition program acknowledges the hard work those working at the bedside do every day, and it comes from their peers. The total cost of this program is $49. Costs include:

- ➢ $4 for the gold can of spray paint
- ➢ $20 for centerpieces
- ➢ $25 for door prizes

Yet, the rewards are endless.

Creative Freethinking

Helping Hands

Once you start to change the culture to achieve the ultimate working experience you will start to see signs of creative freethinking. Motivation + Empowerment = Caregiver Engagement! Empowering those who will benefit the most from the success of each program motivates them to ensure that they are fun and successful. The pure staff engagement then lends itself to the creative thinking process for which many of these programs originate.

A great example of this is the Helping Hands project. This project was created by the Colleague Engagement Committee to help colleagues who fall on hard times. Understanding that people get hungry during the day, the committee bought a box and filled it with lots of candy. The decision was to sell the same things that the vending machines were selling but instead of charging $1.10, they would charge $1.00. Not only are they good at what they do clinically, but they are financially savvy as well. They also provided things that the vending machine didn't have, like healthy selections. All of the proceeds benefit colleagues who needed help. The Colleague Engagement Committee must approve the spending of fund money.

Originally the box was only open to the ED staff. But then others in the hospital heard that it was cheaper to buy candy in the ED than it was to go to the vending machine. They, too started to come to the ER to buy their snacks. Three months later the fund had raised over $4000. Creative freethinking!

Whose Tattoo is Whose

Have you ever been asked to bring in a baby picture, prom photo, or wedding picture so that it could be pinned it to a corkboard for others to figure out who is who? Fun idea, but it's been done a thousand times according to the Colleague Engagement Committee. We needed to make it better! So, they came up with the "Whose tattoo is whose" contest.

One person on the committee, sworn to secrecy, took close-up pictures of various caregivers' tattoos and posted them on the memo board. The ideas was to match the tattoo to the person it belonged to. After I got past the humiliation of rolling up my shirt so that they could take a picture of my tattoo, I quickly grabbed a contest form and got to guessing. It was great fun and a little frightening to see some of the tattoos and know whose bodies they were on.

When staff start to become truly engaged, they do amazing things. They become creative, proactively find solutions to problems and provide excellent care to their patients. With every successful program initiated, comes enthusiasm, engagement, motivation, and the belief in the vision we all set out to obtain. Each success energizes the team to take on the next challenge. No more silos, just one unified team working together toward one common vision.

Game Plan Tip: Inspiring Creative Solutions

So, how do you get a group of individuals to work together and find creative solutions to issues? It takes patience and someone who can stay organized. The following chronological steps can help teams come up with new ideas to help create the best working experience for the caregivers.

1. Clearly identify the issue that you are trying to improve. Get everyone on the same page. As a leader, identify the issue and do not make suggestions on how to improve. Leave it open to interpretation.

2. After the issue has been identified, ask each member of the committee to write down on an index card where they see the roadblocks to success and one creative and fun way to fix it. Ask them to do this without showing the others.

3. As a group, collect the cards and then read each idea out loud one at a time. Brainstorm how to make each idea better. This stimulates conversation and creativity. Remember, no statement is stupid, and if you don't use an idea as a whole you may be able to use a part of it and combine with other ideas.

4. Compare the ideas to some best practices by searching the internet or posting your issues or ideas on professional listservs.

5. Ask friends and family members who are not in healthcare how they would handle the issue. A solution to a healthcare problem can be found in industries not related to healthcare.

For example, Disney's FastPass line is a great way to improve the waiting times for popular rides. Disney identified customer frustrations about the length of time it took in line to ride some of their most popular rides. To help with this, Disney developed a fast pass system where customers could obtain a ticket at 10am for a ride at 12 noon. Anyone possessing one of these FastPass tickets go through the FastPass line and have a much shorter wait.

Recently, hospitals have started using a program similar to this, where patients, from the comfort of their home, can choose a time to arrive at the ER to receive care for their minor illness or injury. Obviously, it is used for lower acuity patients, but wouldn't it be nice to know that when you arrive you will be seen right away? This is a convenience for the patient and helps the hospital keep the flow of patients moving.

CHAPTER 8
MIRROR, MIRROR ON THE WALL

We have discussed engaging the caregivers throughout the majority of this book. I have always believed that before you can create the best patient experience, you must first focus on the caregivers providing that care. Engagement provides the optimal incentive to create a positive patient experience. However, there is one person that you need to take care of before you focus your attention on your staff, and that is you. We are often so focused on making change happen that we are absorbed into the enormity of it all, and we forget to take care of ourselves.

TAKING CARE OF YOU

So many people that have gone into leadership either exit quickly or burn out along the way. I'm often asked, "How do you not take work home with you?" Not the physical projects or paperwork, but the emotional and mental stress that each leader faces every day. I always tell them that it takes practice, but it's a skill that is more important than any other. Leadership stress can consume you. The pressure of it all can cause mental and physical stress. Don't let that happen. Balance between work and life is needed. It's how I'm able to smile every day to go to work and continue to do so when I leave.

Don't Take It Home with You

Let's be clear. This is not an easy thing to do. Some find it easier, but I believe all leaders struggle with balance at some point in their careers. If you're in a leadership role, you most likely have an electronic leash, like a cell phone or a pager, which follows you when you leave work. So leaving it behind can sometimes be a challenge.

There are a few ways to ensure that your leadership challenges don't become your life's torment. First, learn not to take it home with you. My solution, and I admit it is a relatively simple answer, is to do your best when you are at work. Leave nothing on the table. Organize your day, and get done as much as you can in the time frame that is allotted. Write down anything you don't complete. This will help alleviate anxiety from worrying whether or not you will forget to complete a task due the next day.

When I leave at the end of the day, I allow myself to go into home mode. I did this early in my leadership career. There are only so many hours in the day. So, I am constantly asking myself, "Did I give it my all while I was there?" The answer is almost always yes. If that is the case, then I can leave work with a clear conscience.

Just to the left of my office door is a mirror. Yes, I do use that mirror for practical reasons like checking to make sure that there is no spinach stuck between my teeth or to make sure that my head didn't develop hair horns because I had been grabbing it all day as I grapple with the challenges of modern healthcare. That mirror also has a more symbolic meaning to me. As I leave my office each day I look into the mirror, and I again ask myself if I did the best job possible. No one is present with me when I take a final look as I walk out the door. No one is there to convince or lie to me, just me and my mirror. And, if I can truly say yes to that question then I leave the work at work.

If you are unable to use my symbolic mirror idea, it's okay. Leadership is difficult and each individual has to find what works for them. Below you will find other ideas to assist you through your day and provide you with the mental fortitude to leave work at work.

- *Always remember that no leader is perfect.* Mistakes and poor judgments will happen. It is part of leadership. Don't get down on yourself. Instead, look at it as an opportunity for improvement.
- *Find a hobby!* If you rely on your type A personality to shut down your work brain without any type of distraction, you may be asking too much. Distraction creates a positive mental break from the workday. Your hobby could be exercise, photography, or simply

socializing with friends. Work will still be there tomorrow. Trust me.

- *Prioritize.* We talked about keeping a list of tasks on your desk for the next day. I like to take that one step further and before I leave I take that list and I organize it in priority order. This is easier to do on a computer app like Wunderlist where you can easily rearrange the tasks. Either way, find a method to write everything down and prioritize.

- *Find a trusted colleague at work that you can talk to if you need to discuss an issue that is bothering you.* Do it behind closed doors and be sure to be discreet. Maybe have a standing weekly "cleansing" session with other colleagues who understand and empathize with your challenges. Take a few minutes to discuss it, and maybe you can put it to bed until the next day when you actually have the ability to do something about it.

Leadership is an Attitude

I often see leaders who forget why they do what they do. Leadership isn't for everyone, and there is certainly no shame in admitting that to yourself. I compare leadership to marriage. You have to work hard each and every day to maintain a sense of balance and find your happiness. Reinvent a long standing process and make it better. Challenge yourself and volunteer to chair a new committee or take on a program that perhaps you know little about but have developed an interest in doing.

For example, after the shooting in the ED occurred, I struggled to find meaning in my job. The hospital had decided to research different self-defense and de-escalation programs to help protect the bedside caregivers from future acts of violence. Feeling disengaged and uninspired, I decided to volunteer to become an instructor in the program that was chosen in order to feel some sense of purpose after a tragic event. I found that assisting with the search, an area for which I had very little experience, but highly valued its purpose, helped to inspire me at a time when I was trying to find real purpose in what I was doing. I became an instructor and then certified others in the hospital. Whatever it takes to find the true meaning of happiness in the work place. Don't become complacent. Surround yourself with great people who push you to be more than you thought you could be.

What Makes You Happy?

In anything that we do, including our professions, we should be seeking out what makes us happy. Happiness, however, is relative. What makes one person happy may drive another crazy. It is important for leaders to define what it is that makes them happy. That includes asking yourself if you are happy being a leader. I say to caregivers all the time that if you are not happy doing what you are doing, then do something else. That is the beautiful thing about healthcare, there are so many different ways to practice medicine. I encourage them to seek out different opportunities, even if that means needing to leave the department.

So, are you happy being a leader? Do you feel professionally fulfilled? When I asked myself that question, I discovered that I like doing what I do. I enjoy being a leader and, more specifically, I enjoy finding new ways of doing old things. The phrase "Well, that's the way we've always done it" drives me nuts. If there's one thing I have learned from my past mentors, it is that you should never be satisfied with the good, celebrate it, but then push yourself to stretch beyond good and exceed the expectations. Doing this is what motivates me and makes me happy. My staff knows it, and they too accept the challenge to be the best at whatever we do. Working together as a team, we always try to exceed expectations. Engagement at its best.

Managing Your Own Expectations

Dealing with the pressures of leadership on a daily basis can be an exhausting process. You have made a decision and corrected a problem only to find that another problem presents itself. This in its own right can help convince a leader that this profession is not for them. How then do you cope with these overwhelming pressures? How do you avoid giving into the negativity? My thought is don't run from it; instead, embrace it. When I go to work, I always start my day with the same thought, *I will be presented with 10 problems that require my leadership today.* That's right. I eagerly anticipate those issues. Why? How many times have you showed up to work and get hit immediately with an issue as you walk through the door? Accepting this reality can mentally set the tone of your day. By preparing yourself for probable issues that may happen, you give yourself the chance to maintain a better attitude if they do. This mindset can help you avoid the feeling of being overwhelmed. And, if you get less than 10 in a day, you can now look at that as being a good day.

Monitoring Self-engagement

I have been in leadership for a long time now, and I find myself learning new things on a regular basis. Those leaders who believe there is no more to learn should also realize that it's time to give up leadership. It is my internal motivation that drives me to seek out that new knowledge which in turn challenges me and keeps me happy. That is the type of attitude that makes you successful as a leader. Never be satisfied with the status quo. Instead, find ways to extend beyond the expectation of others and of yourself.

Education comes in many forms. Some are veracious readers while others (like me) tend to learn more from the spoken word. Webinars, professional conferences, and workshops help to educate on best practices and provide hands on experience. Knowing what method is best for you is important. There are times when a formal education process is not the way we learn lessons. I believe that over half of the knowledge I have today did not come from a book, but, instead, came from real life experiences. Some of the best lessons are taught the hard way, by making mistakes. In my opinion, you are more likely to learn from a mistake because you are fearful of not making the same mistake twice. That fear is a negative motivation but for a good reason.

One of these life lessons occurred early in my career. I had an assignment of 7 patients working on a telemetry unit. We were short that day, and everyone needed to step up and take extra patients. Angry and overwhelmed, I rushed through my shift. I found as many shortcuts as I could, and skipped the things I thought I could get away with.

As I approached the end of the shift, I had one task to complete, giving out the meds. I remember the pit in my stomach when I realized that in my rush I gave 30 units of regular insulin instead of the 30 units of 70/30 that was ordered. My stomach dropped, and I began to sweat. I dreaded calling the attending physician to tell him. I survived that day, but I never made another medication mistake again in my career. That experience was my greatest teacher.

Game Plan Tip: The Look Back Book

So often we are forced to forge ahead and try to find the next best practice or achieve an even higher score. Although this never-ending pursuit of perfection is a goal we should all strive to meet, we shouldn't do it blindly without looking back at our successes and the way things "used to be." The Look Back Book is a leadership journal of sorts, and one self-engagement method I use. It includes memories of things you changed, accomplishments that you made, and goals that you have exceeded. Snapshots of pass successes allow you, even if it is just for a few minutes, to look back and say, "Wow, look how far we've come!"

Step 1: Use a notebook—or better yet, create a shared file on the intranet—and record each achievement the unit accomplishes. Do this online so that others can enjoy looking back as well.

Step 2: Use the book as a fun fact dictionary for your huggles. When staff morale is low, use the book to show them how successful you've all been as a group and help them enjoy where you are today.

Step 3: The book could even be used to self-motivate when you get tired of your boss constantly asking for more and barely recognizing what already has been accomplished.

Step 4: Use the book and compare notes with your support group. You know, the group of other managers who you sit with behind closed doors and have therapy sessions, having conversations that are more for your peace of mind then for an actual purpose. Don't be embarrassed. We all need these kinds of meetings.

After you have a collection of success stories, you can use them in a variety of ways. At our annual awards banquet, we use the Look Back Book to create a slide show. Each year, we also collect pictures with the stories. As the year winds down, we used the slide show at our annual Golden Urinals awards banquet. After 5 years, we took a look back at all 5 years in one slide show, which made it a fun way to remember good times and old friends who had moved on to other jobs or careers.

Creating Your Own Game Plan

In leadership, there are those who have chosen to follow us. This includes other leaders, and it is one of leadership's greatest responsibilities to be a good mentor and coach for others. I've had leaders ask me to help them take a group of individuals and convert them into a unified, engaged team. I sit down and discuss what they feel are their issues. I do some research and then create a plan specifically catered to the unit. We use many of the techniques and programs described in this book. We set up a chronological "to do" list based on perceived and real roadblocks and present expected outcomes. Inevitably, they look at the time frame for expected improvement and become disheartened. "It's really going take that long?" Yes, it really is, and it's going to be hard work. You're going to have to be persistent, and there will be setbacks that will test your mental fortitude and make you question why you even chose to do this to yourself. Remember, it didn't get this bad overnight, so don't expect it to improve overnight. Have faith!

SEEING THE ENGAGEMENT

This book has been about the process that leaders must go through in order to create the best working experience for caregivers as well as for themselves. How do you know when you truly have achieved staff engagement? Is there a sign? Remember, culture change takes time and sometimes leaders are impatient. But, somewhere along the way, you want that definitive answer to the question: "Have we achieved the vision and culture that we set out to achieve?" The answer is never black and white, but there are telltale signs that you have met your goal. Understanding how to read these signs will encourage you as a leader and help you sustain your own motivation throughout the process.

Reading the Signs: Putting Patients First

One of the most reliable signs that culture change is really happening is when the caregivers find ways to create an experience for their patients not based on a preconceived leadership driven program but from a sense of internal motivation. When they go beyond the diagnosis and find a way to celebrate the human being in that bed. An example of this occurred one morning in our busy emergency room when a patient was placed on a stretcher, which was located around the nurse's station. He was demented and very loud. We were unable to place him into a room because they were all filled.

The patient was confused, thinking that he was at a Philadelphia Eagles game, and he would root loudly when his team would score and scream obscenities at the other team when they had the ball. A few complained, while others walked by the patient without acknowledging that he might need their help. Understanding that this was not his fault, our unit clerk decided that she would try to help this patient. She went to his stretcher and sat next to it. In a calm voice, she asked the patient why he was screaming. Still confused, he stated that his team was losing and kept yelling. Frustrated but unwilling to give up, she decided to try a new approach. She got close to his ear and started softly singing the Philadelphia Eagles fight song, "Fly, Eagles Fly on the road to victory". The patient started to sing along and in a low tone, they sung together. The patient stopped yelling, and peace was restored. She made the human connection because it was the right thing to do.

Reading the Signs: Holding Each Other Accountable

A leader can sometimes feel isolated when it is their sole responsibility to hold others accountable. In the beginning, caregiver engagement can be a daunting task. Be patient. As the culture changes and the caregivers see that your words match your actions, they will start to believe. The positive caregivers will feel empowered and energized. As the culture shifts to one that focuses on the positive working experience each caregiver desires, they will start to take that responsibility on themselves holding each other accountable. I have seen this happen in many ways. I am still always excited to watch an employee march another over to the Clinical Excellence Commitment board, ask them which standard they believe they just violated, ask them to show them where they signed the board, and then ask them to apologize because that is not what they agreed to when they signed it! Engaged employees working together to ensure the best working experience possible has been the goal of this book.

Reading the Signs: Initiating Ideas

Another powerful sign that culture is changing is when staff start coming to you with ideas before you present them with an issue. In other words, they are proactively identifying opportunities for improvement and recommending some action without prompting. This is where true engagement becomes a reality. We said in the beginning that people will want to follow you if they believe in the vision and if they believe in you. As culture changes, so does the investment each caregiver dedicates to the success of the department. Work hard and keep focused as a group. Empower and find ways to motivate those that work at the bedside and true staff engagement can be your reality as well.

Reading the Signs: Treat Each Other Like Family

If you think about it, we spend a lot of our lives at work. Twelve-hour shifts and 40-hour work weeks are all part of our everyday lives. When you spend that much time together, you tend to share moments of your life with those who surround you in the work place. We celebrate joyous occasions, we support each other during difficult times, and we give hugs when tragedies occur. When you see everyone participating in the Helping Hands program so that when the need presents itself there are ways to help out their fellow caregivers, that's engagement. When you witness employees donating their own vacation time to another caregiver when they are suddenly diagnosed with cancer, that's engagement.

I felt the love and support of my colleagues when the shooting occurred in 2005. I could see it in their faces, and I could feel it in my heart. It is a moment that I will never forget, not just because it was an awful thing to happen, but because of the tremendous sense of pride I had as a leader, watching this group of emotionally wounded individuals work together in the face of violence for the benefit of their patients. Their faces filled with panic, but their bodies were totally focused on what had to be done. Truly inspiring.

As I think back on that tragic night, I was proud, and for a split second, I remember saying to myself, *This is the culture that we have been working so hard to achieve.* The support, the focus, the love that was felt that night made it evident that our culture had changed, that we were more than employees, that we were caregivers, to the patients and families that we treated, as well as the people we worked with side by side every day.

REFERENCES

Affordable Care Act Update: Implementing Medicare Cost Savings. Retrieved March 15, 2015, from 0.

AHRQ. (2012). Project Red: Reengineering the discharge process. Retrieved May 2, 2015, from https://cahps.ahrq.gov/surveys-guidance/hospital/hcahps_slide_sets/project_red/projectredtranscript.html.

As Medicare and Medicaid Turn 50, Use of Private Health Plans Surges. Retrieved August 7, 2015, from http://www.nytimes.com/2015/07/30/us/as-medicare-and-medicaid-turn-50-use-of-private-health-plans-surges.html.

Atchinson, T. (2004). Followership: A practical guide to aligning leaders and followers. Chicago, Il: Heath Administration Press.

Obamacare Facts. (2015, August 1). Retrieved August 1, 2015, from http://obamacarefacts.com/sign-ups/obamacare-enrollment-numbers/.

Autry, J.A., (2001). *The Servant Leader: How to build a creative team, develop great morale, and improve bottom-line performance.* New York, NY: Three Rivers Press.

Brehem, S.S., & Brehem, J.W. Reactance theory (1981). Psychological reactance: A theory of freedom and control. New York, NY. Academic Press.

Chick-fil-A. (2014). Company fact sheet. Retrieved July 6, 2015, from http://www.chick-fil-a.com/Company/Highlights-Fact-Sheets.

Collins, J. (2001). *Good to Great: Why some companies make the leap...and others don't.* New York, NY: Harper Collins.

Communication: Fundamental Skills. (2010). Retrieved December 20, 2013, from https://www.mheducation.co.uk/openup/chapters/9780335237487.pdf

Cutting, A.L., & Dunn, J. (1999). Theory of mind, emotional understanding, language, and family background: Individual differences and interrelations. Child Development, 70(4), 853-865.

Goleman, D. (1995). Emotional intelligence: Why it can matter more than IQ. New York: Bantam.

The Huffington Post (2012, April 7). Retrieved July 20, 2015, from http://www.huffingtonpost.com/2012/04/17/hospital-credit-downgrade_n_1431582.html.

Judge, T.A., Piccolo, R.F., Podsakoff, N.P., Shaw, J.C., Rich, B.L. (2010). The relationship between pay and job satisfaction: A meta analysis of the literature. Journal of Vocational Behavior, 77(2). 157-167.

Kotter, J. (2012). Leading Change (1st ed). Boston, MA: Harvard Business School Press.

Mehrabian, A. (1971). Silent messages. Belmont, CA: Wadsworth.

National Patient Safety Foundation & Patient and Family Advisory Council (2000). National agenda for action: Patients and families in patient safety; Nothing about me, without me. Retrieved August 26, 2015, from http://c.ymcdn.com/sites/www.npsf.org/resource/collection/ABAB3CA 8-4E0A-41C5-A480-6DE8B793536C/Nothing_About_Me.pdf.

Russel, J.A., & Bullock, M. (1986). On the dimensions preschoolers use to interpret facial expressions of emotion. Developmental Psychology, 22, 97-102.

Ryan, R.M., & Deci, E.L. (2000). Self-Determination Theory and the Facilitation of Intrinsic Motivation, Social Development, and Well-Being. American Psychologists, 55(1), 68-78.

Spence-Laschinger, H. K., Almost, J., Tuer-Hodes, D., (2003). Workplace empowerment and magnet hospital characteristics making the link. JONA,

33(7/8), 410-422.

State of the American Workplace. (2013). Retrieved February 2, 2015, from http://employeeengagement.com/wp-content/uploads/2013/06/Gallup-2013-State-of-the-American-Workplace-Report.pdf.

Tiered Insurance Networks: Complicating Obamacare or Controlling Costs? Retrieved March 15, 2015, from http://www.cfah.org/blog/2014/tiered-insurance-networks-complicating-obamacare-or-controlling-costs.

Wahba, M.A., (1976). Maslow reconsidered: A review of research on the need hierarchy theory. Organizational Behavior & Human Performance. 15. 212-240.

8 Tips to Help Managers and Employees Deal With Organizational Change. (2010). Retrieved May 10, 2015, from http://www.peterstark.com/managers-employees-organizational-change.

ABOUT THE AUTHOR

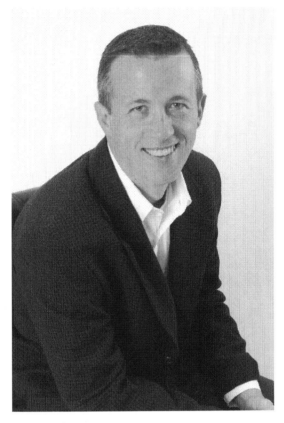

With over 24 years of experience, Charles Kunkle, RN, MSN, CEN, NEA-BC, has held multiple positions in leadership, emergency medicine, prehospital emergency medical services, and cardiothoracic intensive care, having honed his skills over the years as a flight nurse at Boston Medflight.

Charles was named nurse manager of the year by *Nursing Spectrum* magazine in 2006 and was featured in RN Magazine in 2007. A contributing editor and author for Lippincott Publishers, he has been involved in many publications and books.

In 2009, he launched his leadership coaching and consulting firm, Navigator Leadership. His workshops and presentations focus on nurturing staff engagement through motivation, empowerment, and the art of having fun.

As a motivational speaker, Kunkle uses humor, storytelling, and life experiences to captivate audiences while discussing topics such as caregiver engagement, patient experience, emotional intelligence, critical thinking, and creating positive patient experiences. His message has been received by physicians, leaders and, of course, bedside caregivers.

For more information about Charles Kunkle or Navigator Leadership, go to:

http://www.notimetocare.com/
(267) 209-0044

The Entrepreneur's Publisher

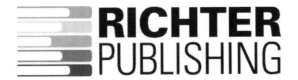

Made in the USA
Charleston, SC
16 February 2016